# Give It To Me Straight!

QUESTIONS & ANSWERS FOR NO-NONSENSE NUTRITION

KIM DALZELL, PHD, RD, LD

*NutriQuest Press*
*Round Lake, Illinois*

**You can order this book from BookMasters, Inc.: 800 247-6553**

IMPORTANT NOTICE TO READERS!

*The information in this book is based upon the latest scientific findings and the personal and professional experiences of the author. The advice given is not intended as a substitute for consulting with your physician or other health care provider. The publisher and author are not responsible for any adverse effects or consequences resulting from the use of any of the suggestions or products discussed in this book. All matters pertaining to your health should be supervised by a qualified health care professional.*

*While the author has made every effort to provide accurate telephone numbers and Internet addresses at the time of publication, neither the publisher nor the author assume any responsibility for errors, or for changes that occur after publication.*

Library of Congress Control Number: 2003096465

ISBN: 0-9712558-2-2

Illustrated by: Steve Ferchaud

Book Design by: Janice M. Phelps

Edited by: Larry Cuba

Back Cover Photo: Fedler Studios

PRINTED IN THE UNITED STATES OF AMERICA

*This book is dedicated to those who ask, and ask again,*
*until they are confident about the answer;*
*and to David and Kathryn, who ask the toughest questions of all!*

## To My Readers,

I think most of us would agree that good nutrition is the foundation for building and maintaining a healthy body. Food can provide you with energy and help you heal, or it can make you sick and miserable. The fact is, you're going to invest a lot of money, time and effort shaping your health for better or worse, so the real question is: where do you want to spend your time—in the produce section or in the hospital?

Redirecting your diet toward prevention will pay off far more than you might think. And the alternative—mounting medical bills, missed employment income, time away from friends and family, and personal pain and suffering—serves only to rob you of precious opportunities and memories. Even if you've been diagnosed with a chronic disease, there is still time to make dietary changes that can boost immunity, promote healing, and significantly impact your quality and quantity of life!

As an oncology nutritionist, professional speaker and nutritional consultant, I answer thousands of inquiries from people all over the world who ask for my advice. Health-conscious consumers want to know what they can do nutritionally to prevent or fight chronic health problems like heart disease or cancer. When I respond to emails, phone calls or raised hands, I hear the same questions repeated, bringing me to the unfortunate conclusion that the basic facts about good nutrition continue to mystify most people. And I can see why! Much of the information aimed at educating and motivating is contradictory and confusing. I'm sure you know what I'm talking about—you pick up an article touting the health benefits of soy and then hear a radio guest questioning soy's health potential. It's enough to make you scream, "What is the right answer?" Wading through all of the clever marketing schemes and latest nutritional breakthroughs doesn't necessarily give you the proper ammunition to change your dietary habits, especially if the advice isn't straightforward or practical. You have to understand the information and integrate it into your life before any real, positive changes occur.

Taking personal responsibility for your health involves more than reading about the latest medical breakthrough or discussing promising new nutrition studies—these actions do nothing more than qualify you as an armchair health nut. Just knowing about healthy choices won't promote wellness or protect you against disease any more than learning about Lance Armstrong will help you win the Tour de France. You must act upon what you know—read product labels, choose foods that are close to nature, and spend more time in the kitchen cooking healthier meals. Taking action can help you achieve greater health, but how can you make sure your actions are based on the best nutritional choices? Read this book!

*Give It To Me Straight! Questions & Answers for No-Nonsense Nutrition* compiles the most frequently asked questions I've received over the past several years and provides answers I feel could help people make better nutritional choices for themselves and for the people they care about. All of the topics I've included are relevant to preventing or fighting cancer and other chronic diseases. Even those interested in general healthy eating will benefit from the practical suggestions! This book will help you gain more control over your health by providing you with solid facts about healthy nutrition and advice on how to make important nutritional and behavioral changes that can make a real difference. And that's just the start! Many answers will provide you with practical tips or product suggestions to help you eat smarter, reduce your health risks, avoid the dangers of "miracle cures" and develop a stronger and healthier body.

I know people want straight answers to their nutrition questions so I've tried to make this book free from scientific or medical rhetoric and as useful and reader-friendly as possible. The special features—called Best Bites—will provide you with practical, shopper-savvy advice so that you can easily put into action what you've learned. I expect that after reading some of the questions in this book you'll respond just as I did: "That's a good question!" And after reading the answers, I hope you'll think, "Now that makes sense!"

The best news is that this book will provide you with enough knowledge that the next time you read about the latest nutrition trend, you'll be in a better position to evaluate its true health potential. You will have learned the basic nutrition facts that will help you make an informed decision for yourself.

I hope you enjoy reading my book and learning about the healing powers of nutrition. Remember, you are worth every good choice you make!

*"Chews" wisely,*
*Kim*

# The Bitter Truth

**Q:** *Is it true that you have to eat the right proportions of acid and alkaline foods for your body to achieve a healthy pH?*

**A:** Your diet can impact pH, but to a much lesser degree than you might think. The kidneys, lungs and internal buffer systems are primarily responsible for making sure you stay in balance. They work together to help rid the body of excess acid produced by normal metabolic functions. Through these mechanisms, you can maintain a health-promoting neutral pH of just above 7.0.

Choosing your foods wisely may also help. Fruits and vegetables provide the body with alkaline mineral buffers that support a neutral environment, whereas highly processed, meals-on-the-run tend to produce additional acid for your system to contend with. Your body just has to work harder to achieve balance.

Proponents of the alkaline diet, which consists of 80% alkaline and 20% acidic foods, believe that if your internal mechanisms are compromised or overworked because of a highly acidic diet, you'll have more difficulty maintaining a healthy pH and you'll increase your risk for disease. Interestingly enough, many disease conditions like cancer, rheumatoid arthritis and chronic fatigue appear to be helped by keeping pH at optimal levels; so I think in terms of disease prevention or progression, it's generally a good idea to eat a more alkaline diet.

While it might be helpful and interesting to look at an acid/alkaline food chart, there's no need to restrict any foods that you know are healthy even if they are listed as acid producing. High acid foods like rye, oat bran, soy milk, peas, carrots and cranberries have health-promoting nutrients and plant chemicals that you don't want to miss out on! If you want to support a neutral environment, cut back on foods that produce the most acid—fried foods, meat, cheese and sugar. It will also help if you avoid alcohol and limit your caffeine intake. Moving toward a diet of unprocessed, whole foods that is rich in fruits and vegetables will help you maintain a healthy pH and support your innate healing potential. As for pH urine test strips, be aware that urine pH is not as rigidly controlled as blood pH, and results can be affected by a number of factors, including the use of certain medications.

## Are you sour on grapefruit?

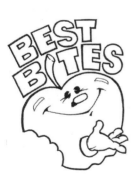

**Many people avoid citrus because they think it's too acidic. But actually, many citrus fruits like grapefruit and oranges break down in the body to an alkaline residue. So while grapefruit tastes acidic, it actually counterbalances acid byproducts and contributes to a health-promoting neutral environment!**

Other foods that alkalinize the body....
Radishes • Cauliflower • Onions • Tangerines
Raisins • Lemons • Strawberries

*Are you surprised?*

# Itching for an Apple?

**Q**: *How can I tell if I have a food allergy?*

**A:** In a true food allergy, the allergen (the most common ones include nuts, milk, eggs, fish, shellfish, soybeans, and wheat) triggers the release of histamines that cause sneezing, sniffling, and localized swelling. If the allergic reaction is severe, anaphylaxis occurs—a life-threatening reaction where the throat tightens and blood pressure drops quickly. You should contact an allergist for a prescription of injectible epinephrine if you develop severe food allergies that might put you at risk for anaphylactic shock.

Many people have minor food intolerances or sensitivities. Although troublesome, these are not true allergic reactions and are usually due to a person's inability to digest a certain food. For example, a lactose-intolerant person doesn't produce enough of the enzyme lactase to properly digest milk sugar. Sometimes cancer treatment can cause temporary lactose intolerance because many of the digestive enzymes have been destroyed by chemotherapy or radiation. Food additives like sulfites (found in wine and dried fruits), monosodium glutamate (found in Chinese food), food colorings, and chocolate and other caffeinated products may also cause reactions in susceptible individuals.

Sometimes you can outgrow a food allergy; but if you don't, you'll probably just have to avoid the offending food because there isn't a treatment or cure for food allergies. If you suspect that you have food allergies, talk with an allergist or immunologist and get tested for food hypersensitivities. Because poorly digested proteins are the culprits behind many food intolerances, digestive enzymes and betaine hydrochloride may help you digest proteins more thoroughly. Complete digestion is especially important for individuals who have compromised immune systems because partially digested proteins can further impair immunity.

Avoid cross-contamination by obtaining a list of foods and food additives from a registered dietitian so that you can read labels more effectively. Some fruits and vegetables cross-react with pollens, such as birch tree pollen or ragweed. If you're allergic to ragweed, for example, you may end up with an itchy mouth, eyes and runny nose when you eat melons and bananas! This common reaction is called Oral Allergy Syndrome (OAS). The skins of fruits and vegetables contain the most protein, so it can help to remove the peel before you eat raw produce. And, if you cook these cross-reactive plants, you shouldn't experience any symptoms at all.

# Catch a Craving

**Q:** *I just finished my fifth chemotherapy treatment and I've lost interest in eating. I really can't afford to lose any more weight. What can I do to increase my appetite?*

**A:** Tell your loved ones not to bother whipping up a five-course gourmet meal for you (in fact, you may want to show them this so they'll stop trying to force feed you!). If you don't feel like eating, mounds of sumptuous food won't tempt you. To avoid losing any more weight, you need to act fast. Ask your doctor about prescription medications that can help you regain your desire to eat and recover lost weight. Megace, one of the most commonly used appetite stimulants, can be taken up to four times a day and can promote significant weight gain in malnourished individuals. Most people report increased appetite within just a few days of starting this medication.

Sometimes, cancer treatment or symptoms related to a chronic disease can make you feel depressed, reducing your desire to eat. If you think this might be the case, ask your doctor if prescription medication to treat mild depression can help you.

To avoid filling up too quickly, eat small, frequent meals throughout the day and make sure you eat healthy, higher calorie foods. This way, you'll consume more nutrients in a smaller volume of food. Add healthy calories to your diet by topping cereals with dried fruit and nuts; sprinkling wheat germ on cereals, yogurt and salads; and adding extra virgin olive oil to beans, greens, pasta, potatoes, chicken, and fish.

Limit zero-calorie, low-nutrition liquids like coffee or tea. Instead, quench your thirst with 100% juice or a high calorie, high protein, weight-gain shake. I usually recommend Prosure, which you can order through your local pharmacist. Mass Fuel, available at health food stores, also packs a powerfully caloric punch.

If appetite stimulants, high calorie shakes, and other dietary modifications don't help you maintain or gain weight, you may need advanced nutritional support. Tube or intravenous feeding used as a complementary therapy to basic cancer treatment can decrease the risk of further deterioration, improve your immunity, help you avoid health complications associated with malnutrition, and enhance your quality of life. Talk to your doctor about this option, and don't delay—malnutrition can significantly slow your recovery.

---

# Are you ready for a power-boost shake or smoothie?

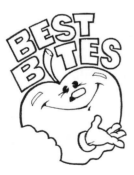

**Try adding ground flax seed, wheat germ, organic yogurt, or powdered milk to your smoothie. You may also want to add a scoop of whey protein powder.**

Available in lots of tasty flavors like chocolate, berry and orange, whey protein boosts the total calories of your drink and contains compounds that help stimulate the immune system.

*Now that's a drink to your health!*

---

# Affection for Confections?

**Q:** *I love sweets but I'm trying to stop eating so much sugar. Should I consume foods that contain artificial sweeteners instead?*

**A:** Cutting back on your sugar intake is always a good move. After all, this white poison can cause dental caries, weight gain, diabetic complications, and immune suppression. But artificial sweeteners are so—artificial! So, what's a sweetaholic to do?

Considering the many low calorie sweeteners on the market today, I would suggest avoiding saccharin and aspartame. Animal studies have shown that saccharin (found in Sweet N'Low) may be a tumor promoter in the bladder, lungs, and other organs. Aspartame, marketed as NutraSweet and Equal, has been linked to neurological disturbances like headaches. Acesulfame K (Sunnet) or sucralose (Splenda) might be suitable substitutes; they have been determined to be safe by regulatory authorities in several countries. You may even want to try the newest addition to the alternative sweetener market—DiabetiSweet, a combination of Acesulfame K and isomalt, an ingredient that adds volume to foods.

While these noncaloric sweeteners may help you cut back your sugar intake, you may not want to consume drinks or food that contain artificial ingredients. A more prudent course of action is to limit your intake of these sweeteners until additional studies confirm long-term consumption safety.

The best choice for people trying to avoid both sugar and artificial sweeteners is Stevia, a more natural alternative to highly refined table sugar. This herbal sweetener is about two hundred times sweeter than sugar, is calorie-free, and comes in liquid and powdered form. Stevia has been shown to effectively lower blood sugar levels—making it a good choice for diabetics and people with hypoglycemia. Stevia's flavor is quite acceptable, although I've received feedback that it has a mild licorice aftertaste. HoneySweet is another natural sweetener. Made from pure honey, this product offers you sweet satisfaction without the heavy industrial processing. You should be able to find Stevia and HoneySweet at your local health food store.

# A Hill of Beans

**Q:** *Why should I eat beans when they make me feel so miserable?*

**A:** If you avoid eating beans because your stomach rebels afterward, don't put down your spoon yet! Beano, an over-the-counter liquid enzyme solution, or health food store digestive enzymes, can help you digest the starches that cause gas. Given the growing body of evidence that beans may effectively defend your body from cancer and heart disease, you should do everything you can to work them into your daily diet.

Packed with vitamins, minerals, and protein, beans are also an excellent source of fiber (10 – 14 grams of fiber per cup). Dietary fiber fills you up, stabilizes blood sugar by providing steady, long-lasting energy, and promotes efficient movement of food through the colon.

Recent studies reveal that populations who eat the most beans have lower rates of cancer of the breast, colon, pancreas, and prostate. Soybeans, in particular, contain special plant hormones that appear to stop the growth of potential cancer cells. Other compounds found in soy may cause cancer cells to become normal or prevent cancer by stopping free radical damage.

Studies show that beans offer cardiac protection as well. Your cholesterol levels can drop by 10% if you eat a cup of beans each day. From adzuki to pinto, beans are chock full of folic acid, a B vitamin that can control levels of homocysteine in the body. Elevated levels of homocysteine contribute to heart disease and can be effectively reduced by the combined actions of folic acid and vitamins B6 and B12.

Ready to eat? Before you cook dried beans, put them in a bowl, pour on plenty of boiling water, and soak overnight. Add a small amount of fat or a protein source like chicken or kombu (a sea vegetable available at Asian markets) to help the beans cook faster and to increase their digestibility, nutrients, and flavor. Of course, if you need a quick meal, just open up a can of beans, heat and eat. Make sure you rinse canned beans with water before using them, because many brands contain tons of sodium. Remember to drink plenty of fluid, too, when introducing these fiber-filled beauties into your diet.

# Any Way You Slice It

Q: *How can I tell if I'm eating nutritious, high-fiber bread?*

A: When you pick up a package of bread, it would seem that you've made a good choice; after all, the United States Department of Agriculture's Food Guide Pyramid recommends six to eleven servings of bread, cereal, rice, and pasta per day—so how can you go wrong?

It can be tricky to wade through marketing claims on packages and find bread that's worth its weight in wheat. Don't be fooled by claims like "made with natural whole grains" or "hearty oats and nuts." Despite the healthy terminology, most grain products contain white flour as the first ingredient. If the label doesn't say 100% whole wheat, chances are the product contains more white than whole grain flour.

Color can be deceiving too. Brown bread is not always better that white bread. In fact, most wheat bread is usually just white bread, with maybe a sprinkling of whole wheat or some caramel coloring to give it a whole grain hue. If you look carefully, you'll find that most rye, pumpernickel, and oatmeal breads are also largely white flour. A number of multigrain breads also contain mostly white flour with a dash of some other grain. Unfortunately, unsuspecting consumers end up eating nutrient-poor, enriched wheat flour products. They lose out on the benefits of the nutrient-packed germ and bran and are supposed to be comforted by the fact that the manufacturer restored just a handful of vitamins and minerals lost during processing!

To qualify as a food that reduces risk of heart disease and cancer, your bread must contain at least 51% whole grain, have a minimum of 1.7 grams of fiber per serving, and be low in fat. And, like any food that carries a health claim, it can't have more than 480 mg of sodium per serving. Smart consumers know to check the serving size as well. Some manufacturers double the serving size to two slices to make their products look like they contain more vitamins, fiber, and protein.

## Best Breads

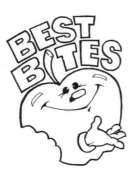

**If you live east of the Mississippi, chances are you've seen (and tasted) Natural Ovens Bakery products on your grocer's bread rack. If you live else-where—I've got good news!**
**You can buy these hearty, whole grain breads online at www.naturalovens.com.**

One of my favorite choices is the Health Max bread—fiber-rich, preservative-free, and full of heart-healthy, immune-stimulating omega-3 fatty acids. You can also find preservative-free, organic Ezekiel bread, made from a variety of sprouted grains, at health food stores.

# Is Butter Still Better?

**Q:** *Are trans-fat-free margarines healthier than butter?*

**A:** Ever since the news hit that butter was better for health than margarine, margarine manufacturers have been racing to formulate better bread spreads. Enter designer spreads like Benecol and Take Care—margarines that have replaced hydrogenated oils or trans fatty acids with sterol esters in an effort to reduce the risk of heart disease. It appears these designer margarines work, too. Studies conclude that six or more pats of the "better spreads" per day have been able to cut LDL (bad cholesterol) by about 15% in people who have high cholesterol levels. Other studies have shown that Enova, a new cooking oil and vegetable spread that blends enzyme-treated soybean and canola oils, helps the body to store less fat and burn it as energy instead.

Beyond issues of health potential and taste preference (many of the patients I've talked to love the buttery flavor of these new spreads), aesthetics might be an issue. While Spectrum Naturals Essential Omega Spread serves up a healthy dose of immune-stimulating omega-3 fatty acids, it may be difficult to get used to seeing a mixture of liquid oil and semisolids when you open the container. It's important to read labels carefully, too, before you choose one of these new margarines. Smart Balance, for example, replaces trans fatty acids with palm oil— a tropical oil that is 50% saturated fat. Even if you eat only a few teaspoons, you're still adding to your overall saturated fat intake. Some companies have added extra calcium or vitamins D and E to their margarines. Although the levels of such additives don't exceed the daily value for any nutrient, if you take dietary supplements, you should be aware of the total levels of nutrients found in your fortified food choices.

There isn't any evidence to suggest that these designer margarines are harmful, but we do know that the spreads can have the undesirable effect of lowering beta-carotene levels. This cancer-protective plant chemical can be found in yellow and orange produce, so as long as you don't exceed the recommended servings of margarine—two to three teaspoons a day—and eat plenty of fruits and vegetables, you should be fine. Beyond reducing total fat intake and minimizing hydrogenated products, other heart-healthy dietary habits include eating more fish and flax, minimizing consumption of refined carbohydrates, eating more soluble-fiber-containing foods like beans, oats, and soy, and enjoying lots of garlic. If you're still not sure which bread spread to buy, just make your own. Mix together a half-cup of butter with a half-cup of extra virgin olive oil. Refrigerate and enjoy in moderation!

# The Hard Facts about Calcium

**Q:** *I'm concerned about getting brittle bones. If I don't drink milk, how can I get my daily requirement of calcium?*

**A:** Milk and milk products are by far the best sources of calcium, but that doesn't mean you can't feed your bones with other foods. Canned fish with edible bones (salmon, sardines, and mackerel) and other plants like kale, broccoli, almonds, and beans are fair sources of calcium. Unfortunately, calcium may not be as available to your body if your diet is high in oxalates (spinach), phytates (whole wheat), protein, or salt.

Bone density increases until age thirty and then gradually declines with age. So if you're younger than that, you've got time to increase your peak bone mass. Even if you're past thirty-five, you can keep your bones strong by consuming a calcium-rich diet and participating in a weight-bearing exercise program.

Many women, especially those who don't like or can't tolerate dairy foods, should take calcium pills as a supplement to their diet. The best-absorbed form of calcium from a pill is calcium carbonate, although seniors tend to absorb the gluconate and citrate forms better. I would recommend avoiding bone meal, dolomite, and oyster shell calcium supplements because they may be contaminated with toxic metals like arsenic, mercury, lead, cadmium, and other heavy metals. I also have some concerns about using antacids as calcium supplements. Antacids tend to decrease the absorption of other vitamins and minerals, like vitamin C, iron, and riboflavin. And, antacids don't contain vitamin D—a nutrient that helps the body absorb calcium. If you have heart, kidney, or liver disease, high blood pressure, primary hyperthyroidism, prostate cancer, sarcoidosis, or multiple myeloma, you should ask your doctor before you begin taking calcium supplements.

Calcium supplement labels typically state that the product provides between 500 and 1,000 mg of calcium; however, the product may actually contain less of the elemental calcium you need than implied on the label. That's because calcium supplements consist of "blends," like calcium carbonate or calcium citrate, which contain roughly 40% and 20% elemental calcium, respectively. These percentages mean that a 1,000 mg calcium supplement may supply only 400 or 200 mg, respectively, of elemental calcium, depending on the form of calcium. The new dietary reference intakes for elemental calcium suggest that adults age nineteen to fifty take 1,000 mg per day and adults over fifty years take 1,200 mg per day. If you take estrogen, you might require less calcium, so ask your doctor for his or her recommendation.

If you have difficulty swallowing calcium pills, carbonate chews, at only 20 calories each, are a great alternative to pills and can offer a sweet ending to your meal. Viactiv Soft Calcium Chews, GNC ActiveCal, and other brands are available in a variety of delicious flavors and contain 400 to 500 mg of calcium each. Find them in the vitamin aisle of your local grocery store.

## Watch out for these dietary calcium zappers!

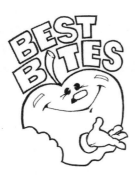

- **Coffee, soft drinks and diuretics**
- **Too much protein, especially meat**
- **Too many concentrated sugars**
- **Alcohol and tobacco**
- **Too little or too much exercise**
- **Too much salt**

# Eat to Prevent Cancer

Q: *Cancer runs in my family. What are some simple tips for changing my diet to reduce my risk of getting cancer?*

A: According to the American Cancer Society and thousands of scientific studies, you can prevent cancer with nutrition—but there is no single food or nutrient that will provide complete protection against the disease. There are a number of dietary guidelines to follow if you want to reduce your chances of developing cancer. As a side benefit, eating right can help you prevent a number of other diseases as well, including heart disease, obesity, and diabetes.

Ease into healthy eating by thinking "plants." Add a fruit or vegetable serving to your diet and work your way to five servings per day. Produce is naturally low in fat and contains plenty of disease-fighting nutrients called phytochemicals. These plant compounds protect cells from free radical damage, inhibit the enzymes responsible for cancer growth, and activate the protective enzymes that stop cancer from progressing. Choose richly colored produce—darker plants contain the most health-protecting chemicals.

You can promote natural detoxification by eating less refined foods and more whole grain foods. Whenever possible, eat brown rice and whole grain breads, cereals, and pastas. Whole grains contain fiber that passes through your body, carrying with it excess estrogen, cancer-causing bile acids, cholesterol, and other compounds that may negatively impact health. The National Cancer Institute recommends you consume between 25 and 35 grams of dietary fiber per day.

By eating a plant-based diet, you not only get the health benefits from the plant nutrients, you also reduce your intake of animal fats. These saturated fats have been linked to a number of cancers. Diets high in saturated fats may also suppress the immune system. Trans fatty acids are abundant in hydrogenated products and are especially unhealthy. To counterbalance the unhealthy fats we eat, it's wise to consume a daily dose of omega-3 fatty acids. Found in cold water fish (salmon, tuna, and mackerel) and flaxseeds, these healthy oils help protect against cancer and heart disease and may offer pain relief for those suffering from rheumatoid arthritis and other inflammatory diseases.

By eating a variety of foods, rich in phytonutrients, fiber, and healthy oils, you can help protect yourself from cancer. While research continues to show that food provides the body with the most effective, health-promoting nutrients, individuals who consistently follow risky dietary practices may benefit from a whole foods nutritional supplementation program. Antioxidant supplements, such as beta carotene, vitamins C and E, and selenium, may also work together with food to provide optimum cancer-fighting protection.

Don't forget to adjust your lifestyle habits: limit alcohol consumption, avoid tobacco, get enough exercise and get off the stress train! The above dietary and lifestyle strategies aren't unrealistic, but they do require time, effort and personal commitment.

# Supplementing Your Cancer Treatment

**Q:** *Is it safe to take dietary supplements if I have cancer?*

**A:** Most conventional cancer doctors insist that patients avoid taking dietary supplements, especially antioxidants, until chemotherapy and radiation treatments have been completed. More than likely they've come to this decision because a handful of studies have suggested that taking antioxidants might decrease the effectiveness of the treatment. For example, studies have shown that N-acetyl cysteine or high doses of vitamin B6 may interfere with cisplatin or other platinum-containing chemotherapies. Additionally, genistein (a soy isoflavone) has been found to compete for estrogen receptors, potentially decreasing the effectiveness of Tamoxifen. However, we have evidence from a large number of research studies to show that dietary supplementation during treatment may offer a variety of benefits, including immune stimulation, cell protection, and detoxification assistance.

Numerous studies suggest that dietary supplements used during cancer treatment can support the whole body during the cancer destruction process and prevent adverse side effects of treatment. For example, a study of breast cancer patients taking CoQ10 during Adriamycin treatment had 20% less heart damage than individuals taking Adriamycin alone. Further supporting the use of dietary supplements during treatment, test tube and animal findings suggest that it isn't counterproductive to take antioxidants—in fact, they may actually enhance treatment outcome. For example, irradiated animals receiving vitamin E before, during and after treatment exhibited lower cancer cell division than did controls, and their normal cells were also protected from damage.

Whether or not you choose to take antioxidants during treatment, as a cancer patient you should remember that you have unique nutritional needs, and that your chances of eating right every day to meet those needs are poor, especially if you are undergoing treatment. If you are a cancer patient, your nutritional and detoxification requirements may also be much higher than a so-called healthy individual's. A cancer patient's rapid cellular turnover rate and greater exposure to damage from chemicals and free radicals point to special nutritional needs. These needs are further supported by evidence that up to 80% of cancer patients develop some degree of malnutrition. If you don't obtain enough nutrients to sustain your body's ever-changing state, it may be difficult to successfully recover your health. A large study in Finland drives home this important point. Cancer patients who had lower levels of selenium and vitamin E had an eleven-fold greater death rate compared to cancer patients who had adequate levels of these nutrients.

I urge you to seek the advice of an oncology nutritionist who can assess your diet to determine if you would benefit from any nutritional supplementation. As always, it is important that you discuss the potential benefits and drawbacks of dietary supplementation with your health care provider.

# Taking Chances with Canola?

Q: *I've heard canola oil might be toxic. Should I avoid it and use olive oil instead?*

A: There's been some bad press circulating about canola oil, probably because it comes from the rape plant, which contains erucic acid—a very toxic and poisonous acid. People who believe that canola oil is toxic cite rat studies that have linked this oil to irreversible fatty degeneration of the heart, kidneys, and other organs. The studies, however, are not widely accepted as proof that canola oil consumption is dangerous. Here's why:

Until 1974, oils made from rapeseed containing up to 40% erucic acid were marketed for human consumption in Canada. After learning of the rat study results, the Canadian government became concerned and worked to develop new varieties of rapeseed containing less than 1% erucic acid. The new oil, called canola (the Canadian oil), was eventually put on the Generally Recognized As Safe (GRAS) list and sold in the United States.

When researchers repeated the rapeseed oil studies with rats, they used sunflower seed oil (which doesn't contain erucic acid). As it turned out, the rats ended up with the same health problems as observed in the earlier studies with rapeseed oil. Scientists concluded that, unlike humans, rats just don't metabolize fats and oils very well and that's why any kind of fat would cause damage to these little creatures!

Today we know that low erucic acid rapeseed oil doesn't harm human hearts and in fact, contains monounsaturated fatty acids that may protect cells from toxic substances. Some people still don't buy canola's safety assurances and argue that it takes years of canola consumption before health problems develop. But if that were true, the Chinese and Indian populations that have used high erucic acid oils for generations would have experienced detrimental effects by now—and they haven't. Note, however, that their oils were not refined or genetically modified (unlike the oils in your supermarket).

Today, about half the canola crop is genetically modified and there's no way to tell if the oil you buy comes from a reengineered plant or not. Refined canola oil may also contain chemical solvent residue and most likely will lack the healthy fatty acids found in unrefined oils. You'd be better off buying organically grown, expeller-pressed canola oil at the health food store or going with the old standby: extra virgin olive oil—unrefined, non-genetically modified, and much less controversial.

# Craving Carbs?

**Q:** *How can I curb my desire for sweets and other high-carbohydrate foods?*

**A:** Can't stop munching on cookies, breads, and other refined carbohydrates? You're not alone! We currently manage to eat nearly 400 calories in sugar every day, causing our blood sugar levels to skyrocket, which in turn, can lead to potential problems with insulin resistance, weight gain and other health concerns. Refined carbohydrates can also feed *Candida albicans,* a yeast infection commonly found in advanced cancer cases, which can cause digestive disturbances and make eating a painful, difficult task.

A number of studies show that in response to hunger we usually reach for something sweet. But once simple sugars are consumed, blood sugar levels rise sharply and then drop, sending signals to the brain that the body needs to be fed again. From this premise, it would appear that controlling blood sugar response is crucial to controlling carbohydrate cravings.

Let the glycemic index (see www.diabetesnet.com for more information) be your guide when choosing carbohydrate foods. This tool will tell you which foods are less likely to cause sharp fluctuations in blood glucose or insulin levels. Beans, whole grains (like rye, oats and barley), nontropical fruits and nonstarchy vegetables (broccoli, spinach and tomatoes) all rate low on the index and thus are good because they take a bit longer for the body to digest and their sugars tend to enter into the bloodstream more slowly. A key point to remember is that if you eat a mixed diet (carbohydrates and protein) you will automatically lower the glycemic index of each meal.

Eat sensibly. Skipping breakfast, for example, can set you up for a mid-morning snack attack. Meal choices should contain a combination of complex carbohydrates (whole grain cereals, breads, and pastas) and proteins (eggs, soy, fish and nuts) to sustain energy levels and support a balanced blood sugar. While it isn't necessary to measure out every ounce of carbohydrate you eat, you do need to eat correct portion sizes. Serving sizes vary by carbohydrate source, so check the package label to give you an idea of how much you should be eating. You may be shocked to learn that a heaping plate of spaghetti may contain over five servings of pasta!

Resist the temptation to follow the popular high protein, low carbohydrate diet programs. The upswing about these diets is that they motivate people to cut down on sugary foods and eat more brown rice and pasta. Unfortunately, they also shun health-enhancing sweet vegetables like carrots and beets, and fruits, robbing the dieter of valuable plant chemicals that enhance digestion, support detoxification, and protect against cellular oxidation.

Starch blockers, which work by deactivating enzymes that convert starch into glucose and then fat, are the latest approach to carb-control dieting. Short-term studies show they effectively reduce carbohydrate absorption and don't appear to effect vitamin or mineral absorption. However, until we have longer-term safety studies on starch blockers, I would suggest avoiding them and learn how to limit your portion sizes. After all, eventually you will have to practice dietary modification if you want weight loss that lasts.

# Bide your time!

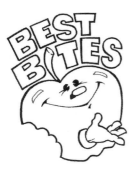

**Most food cravings only last about 10 minutes. So, distract yourself by reading a good book, calling a friend or folding the laundry. Wait and see if the craving passes. If it doesn't, I suggest you go ahead and indulge in a small serving of whatever is calling your name. Better to do it now than to answer the call at midnight!**

*Other helpful hints to help you curb cravings:*
- Walk away from stressful situations
- Meditate regularly
- Cut your desserts in half or replace them with a whole piece of fruit
- Avoid dietary stimulants like coffee or chocolate
- Support adrenal glands with B vitamins, adrenal glandulars and antioxidants

# The Case for Chocolate

**Q:** *Does chocolate really have healthful properties?*

**A:** Chocoholics rejoice! All kinds of chocolate have been used for centuries for healing and pleasure, but dark chocolate seems to have the most to offer when it comes to protecting your health. The latest research suggests that cocoa beans, used to make chocolate bars and other mouthwatering confections, contain health-promoting chemicals.

These chemicals, also found in green tea and a variety of fruits and vegetables, have powerful antioxidant benefits.

According to the Chocolate Information Center (and who wouldn't want to believe them?), people who consume chocolate as part of a balanced diet can potentially reduce their risk of heart disease. Recent published studies back up this health claim. Cocoa plant chemicals called catechins may promote cardiovascular health in a number of ways. For example, studies on humans have shown that cocoa and chocolate consumption reduces inflammation and prevents formation of blood clots. Scientists at the University of California and Mars Company found that cocoa's chemicals relax smooth muscles and promote vascular dilation—both important to maintaining good blood flow through the body. Unsaturated fatty acids found in cocoa butter decrease LDL, or bad cholesterol, according to a study published in the February 2003 issue of the *Journal of the American Dietetic Association*.

Dieters, you too can rejoice! Eating chocolate may help you lose weight. According to an article published in the *Journal of Biological*

*Chemistry,* chocolate contains theobromine, theophylline and caffeine—compounds that send signals to the brain to suppress appetite and create a feeling of fullness. Think about it—you can satisfy hunger pangs by capping off dinner with a chunk of creamy, dark chocolate!

While the news about chocolate may be sweet, you might want to think twice before you dive into a whole box of Godiva chocolates. After all, the American Cocoa Research Institute has funded most of the research on chocolate, and they stand to gain from positive research outcomes. Most importantly, the studies focus on cocoa and don't account for other ingredients found in chocolate bars—fat, sugar, and calories! For now, I'd suggest that you don't toss chocolate in with fruits and vegetables as health-promoting dietary choices. Since the studies show positive health benefits only for just a few hours after cocoa consumption, we need some long-term studies to determine whether or not chocolate is good for our health. I have a feeling that there will be no shortage of volunteers for those studies!

## Deep, Dark and Disease-Fighting!

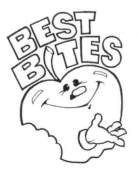

Satisfy your chocolate craving with a piece of dark chocolate, which is lower in sugar and fat that the milk chocolate variety and has more cocoa (and therefore, more health-promoting chemicals).

For a delicious, guilt-free chocolate sauce (courtesy of my editor, Larry): take unsweetened European-style cocoa, mix it with plain soy milk and filtered water, and add a little Stevia for sweetness and vanilla extract for flavor.

# The Right Combination

Q: *Someone told me to try the food combining diet to help lessen my indigestion. Could it really help?*

A: Probably not. I'm always skeptical of diets that encourage severe restrictions of any kind, and food combination diets do just that!

Food combining is based on a theory that different foods require different enzymes for digesting, and eating the wrong combinations of foods will cause digestive disturbances. Most food combining diet plans stipulate that protein and carbohydrate should be consumed at separate times because the acids in protein neutralize the alkaline medium required for digesting the starch in carbohydrates, resulting in fermentation and indigestion. The diet plan also suggests that fat and protein be eaten at separate meals, and that certain foods like nuts (which are 50% fat and can be very difficult to digest) and melons should be eaten separately because they don't combine well with almost any food. Tell that to my fruit salad!

Although a number of food combining diets exist, many begin with a fast of some sort; dieters are instructed to eat only fruit for several days. Thereafter, a small amount of bread and butter is permitted with a few vegetables, and later some meat and shellfish is allowed.

So what's the bottom line? Food combining diets just don't make sense. Your stomach creates a number of digestive enzymes that perform their work on food in the small intestine, with different aspects of digestion occurring along the way. Pancreatic juice is secreted into the small intestine and contains enzymes that digest proteins, carbohydrates, and fats. Our bodies are designed to handle all kinds of foods whenever we choose to eat them.

While food combining diets will help you lose weight (because of the very low calorie nature of the early stages of the diet), weight loss doesn't last because it's difficult to follow this kind of diet for too long. I suggest that if you have a problem digesting food, you try adding digestive enzymes to your nutritional regimen. Remember that whenever you increase your fiber or soy foods intake, you will probably experience more gas and bloating. This is normal and can be alleviated by drinking lots of water and taking digestive enzymes. All in all, the food combining diet appears to be safe, but is unscientific and very regimented. My advice is to avoid the food combining diet and stick with a varied diet—eating right is hard enough without having to follow even more rules!

# The Supplement Secret

**Q:** *Should I tell my doctor if I'm taking dietary supplements?*

**A:** According to a study in the *Journal of the American Medical Association,* more than 80% of American adults take at least one type of medication—from over-the-counter remedies to prescription drugs to dietary supplements. The fact is, many Americans take dietary supplements, and most don't tell their doctors that they use them. Without this information, your doctor may erroneously conclude that your recent complaint of stomach distress, skin rash, or some other side effect is caused by drug intolerance. This misunderstanding could lead to costly changes in medication or discontinued treatment in some instances.

Whether or not your physician approves of your natural therapy approach, you stand a better chance of receiving the best medical care possible when you share all information pertinent to your health. Lack of communication about dietary supplements creates an information gap between health care provider and patient, resulting in poor health management, especially if you are on a number of prescription medications, have a complicated medical history, or are undergoing treatment for a chronic disease.

Taking dietary supplements is not risk free—a variety of nutrients act like drugs; they contain active ingredients that have strong physiological effects. For example, Coumadin, aspirin, omega-3 fatty acids, and gingko biloba all thin the blood, increasing the risk for excessive bleeding. Researchers are finding that many nutrients can be toxic when consumed in large amounts for a period of time, or in combination with other substances. For example, shark cartilage has been linked to several cases of hepatitis, and women taking 5,000 IU of vitamin A may be at increased risk for hip fractures. Keep in mind that manufacturers don't always include safety warnings about potential adverse side effects on the labels of their products. Although your pharmacist can alert you to any drug/nutrient interactions known to exist for your prescription medications, only a limited number of supplements have been researched for their potential interactions with drugs. Ultimately, it is up to you to monitor the safety of your nutrition supplement regimen.

If you develop an upset stomach, dizziness, rash or some other adverse reaction, I suggest that you stop taking all supplements and notify your doctor right away. This action will make it easier for your doctor to determine the cause of your symptoms. You should also check the labels of your supplements to make sure you aren't allergic to any of the ingredients. Once your symptoms are resolved, you should restart your vitamin regimen one supplement at a time, being careful to add no more than one new supplement every two or three days until you determine which supplement may have caused the problem. By the way, you should contact the Food and Drug Administration (FDA) if you experience serious adverse side effects related to the use of dietary supplements. The more the FDA knows about supplement-related side effects, the better they can educate the public about the potential risks associated with using certain nutrients. Call 1-800-FDA-1088 to report your findings.

# Curing Cancer with Calcium?

**Q:** *Should I use coral calcium to fight cancer or prevent other diseases?*

**A:** While coral calcium may be nothing more than a clever marketing gimmick, there is no debating that calcium supplements prevents disease. For example, hundreds of studies have demonstrated the positive effect of calcium supplements on bone health and a recent study in the *American Journal of Medicine* found that postmenopausal women who took 1,000 mg of calcium daily for one year reduced their risk of heart attack by up to 30%. Another study in the *Journal of the National Cancer Institute* revealed that individuals who consumed at least 700 mg of calcium per day (from food and supplements) had about half the risk of developing colon cancer as those getting less than 500 mg daily.

I have a problem with coral calcium because the manufacturers lead people to believe that their calcium, which is extracted from remnants of coral reefs in Okinawa, has unique health properties that prevent and reverse degenerative diseases like cancer, diabetes, heart disease, and more. But coral calcium is not some magical mineral formula—it's simply calcium with some magnesium and other minerals thrown in.

It is true that the people of Okinawa, who supposedly drink water containing coral calcium, live longer and have low rates of heart disease and cancer. But their relatively disease-free life expectancy is most likely due to their activity level and diet, which is rich in plants, soy, fish, and green tea.

Coral calcium is one of several mineral products on the market that supply the body with calcium, but there is no research to suggest that coral calcium does a better job of promoting health than calcium carbonate or calcium citrate (two of the most frequently used forms of supplemental calcium). Furthermore, calcium carbonate (the form of calcium in coral calcium) isn't absorbed by the body as well as calcium citrate. Also be aware that independent laboratory tests have confirmed the presence of lead and other heavy metals in some coral calcium supplements.

Considering all of these facts, I believe you need to ask yourself why you would want to invest in a costly supplement when you can get a safer and more absorbable form of calcium from a local health food store for just cents a day.

# The Cost of Good Nutrition

Q: *Does eating well have to be expensive?*

A: With a bit of planning and time, even if you have a limited income, you can eat healthy. In fact, according to a recent study in the *Journal of the American Dietetic Association,* switching to a diet of mostly low sugar, low fat foods can cut your grocery bill by up to $600 each year!

Foods prepared from ingredients at home are usually less expensive than packaged mixes and frozen entrées, so think, "scratch" instead of "box." The best part about cooking from scratch is that you have control over the ingredients. You can improve your recipes by omitting the salt, reducing the amount of fat or sugar, or substituting whole wheat flour for refined white flour.

As long as storage space isn't an issue, you should buy in bulk. Whether an item is on special or not, bulk purchasing can be less expensive than buying individual serving sizes of food. Fresh fruits and vegetables in season can be far less costly than most packaged snack foods. It makes sense to buy grapefruits, oranges, carrots, and celery in bulk because these kinds of plants tend to have a longer shelf life. If you live alone, you might want to offer to split bags of fresh vegetables or fruit with a neighbor or friend. Peppers, tomatoes, cucumbers, berries, and bananas usually spoil before you get a chance to eat them—sharing them with a friend can help prevent waste.

Main entrées and desserts can be prepared at home, with alterations in fat and sugar content to make them more nutritious. Using less of the more expensive (but less healthful) ingredients can really reduce costs. Add a sprinkling of grated cheese to salads or on top of a casserole or sandwich instead of using it as a main ingredient. Meatless meats (soy dogs, soy "hamburger" crumbles), vegetables, whole grains and legumes that are canned or rehydrated are economical and healthful choices. Healthy snacks like air-popped popcorn, mixtures of dry cereals, seeds and nuts, whole grain muffins, and seasonal fresh fruit can round out your meals and help you meet your food budget and health goals.

You don't have to head to the health food store to shop for organic or otherwise "healthy" foods. Many larger supermarkets have health food specialty aisles, complete with organic canned and packaged products, frozen entrées, and hydrogenation-free snacks. You will typically pay a premium price for these items, so look inside the packages for cents-off or buy-one-get-one-free coupons to use next time you shop. Many of the vegetarian and "health food" companies distribute free consumer newsletters containing coupons, recipe suggestions, and general health information—just call or write to the address on the product label. Coupon clipping, especially for brands that are usually purchased anyway, can shave as much as 10% off food bills. And many stores offer double or triple the face value of the coupon.

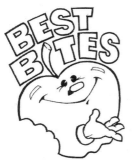

# For free nutrition information, coupons and recipes:

**Organic Valley Farms:**
   1.888.444.6455
**Horizon Organic:**
   www.horizonorganic.com / 1.888.494.3020
**Mambo Sprouts:**
   www.mambosprouts.com
**Eden Foods:**
   1.888.441.3336

# Clotting the Issue

**Q:** *Do I really need to avoid all leafy green vegetables because I'm taking Coumadin?*

**A:** Changes in the amount of vitamin K that you eat can affect the way your Coumadin works. Coumadin, an anticoagulant drug used to prevent blood clots from forming, is given to people who have a history of blood clots, such as those with artificial heart valves, deep vein thrombosis (blood clots in the legs), and certain heart rhythm irregularities such as atrial fibrillation.

Anticoagulants act by blocking the blood-clotting effects of vitamin K, which is abundant in green, leafy vegetables. So, doctors may instruct you to avoid greens and other foods high in vitamin K—they don't want your diet to interfere with the action of the drug. Doctors monitor the effects of the drug by using a routine blood test that measures the clotting time of the blood; they alter the dosage of the drug according to the results of these blood tests. The goal is to keep the clotting time within a relatively narrow range to reduce the risk of bleeding and formation of blood clots.

If you eat a diet high in vitamin K, your blood may get too thick, whereas lowering your vitamin K intake may cause your blood to be too thin. The key is to keep a relatively steady diet so that the amount of vitamin K you eat remains the same. You should be consistent in your intake of dark green, leafy vegetables, broccoli, green tea, lettuce, cabbage, spinach, certain legumes and vegetable oils—they contain the most vitamin K. You may even want to limit the amount of vitamin K-rich foods to one serving per day—but don't avoid them altogether!

Dietary supplements like vitamins A, C and E, flax and fish oil can also alter your blood clotting time. Be careful with "green foods" supplements too. Vitamin K-rich chlorophyll found in green plant dietary supplements, such as barley grass, chlorella and wheat grass, can reduce the effectiveness of Coumadin, especially if your regular diet has previously been low in vitamin K-rich foods.

# Ditch the Decaf?

**Q:** *Is decaf healthier than regular coffee?*

**A:** Put down your coffee cup and listen up! The latest buzz on caffeine is that it may actually be good for you. Researchers reveal coffee drinkers may have a reduced risk for type II diabetes and some cancers. And some doctors are prescribing a cup of Joe for migraine sufferers—caffeine appears to accelerate the pain relieving effects of ibuprofen.

Drinking too much coffee does have its drawbacks though. Excessive caffeine has been linked to bone loss, dehydration, hardening of the arteries, nervousness, and fibrocystic breast disease. Switching to decaf, however, might not be the best solution. Most decaffeinated beverages still retain enough caffeine to affect sensitive individuals. And compounds in coffee other than caffeine may be responsible for its effects on the heart. Case in point: A recent study found that all participants drinking a triple espresso, either with or without caffeine, had blood pressure spikes and increased nervous system activity. Another study found that while regular coffee intake didn't affect the risk for rheumatoid arthritis, women who drank four or more cups of decaf per day doubled their risk of rheumatoid arthritis. Solvents used in the decaffeinating process may also cause health problems, so you may want to look for decaf products that have been water extracted.

Coffee substitutes, made of roasted chicory root, dandelion root and barley, could be the best brew for individuals who want to avoid choosing between regular and decaf. Roastaroma, Cafix, and Pero are popular grain beverages that are available in health food stores and supermarkets.

# Detox Dilemmas

**Q:** *I've just finished chemotherapy; should I go through some sort of detoxification?*

**A:** Because of the potential toxic buildup of medications, exposure to food additives, preservatives, and environmental pollutants, you may benefit from some kind of detoxification in an effort to rid the body of harmful substances. But what kind of detoxification therapy should you do? Our bodies naturally self-cleanse through exhalation, perspiration, urination, and bowel elimination—so if you change your diet, exercise regularly, and reduce the chemicals you put into your body, you should be able to help that detoxification process. Beyond basic diet and lifestyle changes, there are several detoxification therapies that are more advanced but less natural:

Fasting, one of the more uncomplicated therapies, is usually done for a specific number of days in an effort to reduce the amount of toxins coming in so that the body can concentrate on getting accumulated toxins out. Water is always permitted so that dehydration is prevented. People who have problems regulating their blood sugar levels or who are in a weakened state may have difficulty fasting for the required amount of time.

Cleansing of the large intestine with herbal, coffee, or other flushes is called colon therapy. Trained professionals use a tube and nozzle to insert a cleansing solution into the rectum to remove toxic stool buildup. Sometimes an enema is used to clean out the rectum so that colon therapy can be performed more efficiently. Bowel perforation, bacterial infections, and electrolyte imbalances can occur if the procedure is not performed properly.

Chelation therapy has been used to treat heavy metal poisoning (such as mercury or lead) and hardening of the arteries. Patients are infused with a chemical called EDTA, which binds to heavy metals in the blood. The toxic metals are then flushed out naturally through the kidneys. Benefits of chelation therapy might be short-lived if you return to a high fat, chemically laden diet. One of the potential drawbacks of chelation therapy is that excessive chelation treatment can also remove from your body beneficial minerals (such as copper, zinc, manganese, magnesium, and calcium) required for normal metabolic activity.

Before you embark on any of these detoxification therapies, I suggest you seek professional advice and monitoring. I haven't found much data to support the theory that detoxification therapies work, but I've had patients report lowered blood pressure, reduced blood fat levels, enhanced mental clarity, and better digestion after completing a detoxification program.

---

# Detox naturally!

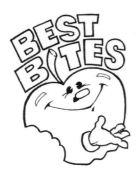

- Drink at least eight, 8- to 12-ounce glasses of fluid each day
- Eat lots of fruits and vegetables
- Bulk up your diet with fiber-rich whole grains and legumes
- Consider adding digestive enzymes to your supplement regimen
- Exercise regularly
- Take a steam bath or sauna
- Get a massage
- Try milk thistle, yellow dock and dandelion supplements.

# Good for the Gut

**Q:** *I seem to have a difficult time digesting certain foods. Can enzymes help?*

**A:** Yes! Our body normally makes and uses a variety of enzymes that help us break down food into basic building blocks so we can then absorb and reassemble nutrients to build cells, tissues organs, glands, and the entire body. Chemotherapy and other medications, certain health conditions or just getting older can affect how our bodies produce enzymes. These factors, coupled with the destructive effects of cooking and processing on live plant enzymes, will leave most people with a shortage of digestive enzymes.

When foods aren't completely digested, we tend to experience a number of uncomfortable symptoms, including bloating, gas, indigestion, acid reflux, heartburn, and other digestive difficulties. Poor digestion can also prevent the absorption of valuable nutrients, causing potential vitamin and mineral deficiencies. Undigested foods can also putrefy in the intestines, feeding undesirable microorganisms that produce harmful gas and toxins. A phenomenon known as leaky gut syndrome—caused by undigested proteins that make their way into the bloodstream and wreak havoc on the immune system—can lead to allergies, autoimmune disorders, inflammation, migraines, skin conditions, respiratory difficulties, behavioral changes, and many other symptoms.

If you think that you have poor digestion, you may want to consider eating more raw and sprouted foods, which contain active plant enzymes, and supplement your diet with digestive enzymes.

Enzymes have no taste, so feel free to open up the capsules and throw the contents into your food (as long as your foods aren't hot!). You may also swallow capsules before or during meals according to the manufacturer's recommendations. Don't worry about overdosing on enzymes; you can use as many enzymes as necessary to optimize digestion. If you have active stomach ulcers, check with your doctor before you take digestive enzymes.

I suggest you buy a plant-derived enzyme supplement. Plant enzymes work in both low- and high-pH environments, so they have a wide range of activity throughout the digestive tract. To better digest carbohydrates, proteins, and fats, take a broad-spectrum supplement that contains amylase, protease, and lipase.

# On your way to digestive wellness:

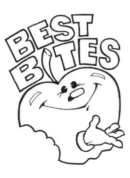

- Eat slowly and relax during mealtimes.
- Gently detoxify with juicing or plant-based diet therapies.
- Eat yogurt or take a probiotic to ensure a balance of healthy gut bacteria.
- Aid digestion by eating raw foods, which contain live enzymes.
- Drink purified water to assist with total body cleansing.
- Respect your individual food intolerances or allergies.

# Fast Fuel

**Q:** *The energy or protein bars that I get at the health food store are delicious, but are they any healthier than a regular candy bar?*

**A:** Energy bars are not for endurance athletes any more; their chewy goodness appeals to everyone. After all, who wouldn't want to indulge in a guilt-free version of a candy bar? The reality, however, is that many of these bars are health food imposters. They tend to be a bit costly, too. Why not spend less money and gain more nutritional value by eating a piece of fruit and a cup of yogurt, or a handful of trail mix?

I believe most people like energy bars because they are an effective substitute for a meal or snack. But before you grab and go, I suggest you carefully read the package label. Many energy bars contain too many calories, fat, sugar, and other ingredients that you might not want to consume. Women with breast cancer or who are on Tamoxifen, for example, will want to check to make sure their bars don't contain isolated soy protein. This concentrated source of soy protein contains high levels of isoflavones that may spur on the growth of hormone-sensitive cancer cells.

Also check the serving size. Some products may contain two or more small bars inside one wrapper, and each small bar may constitute a full serving. It's easy to overlook these extra servings, consume the entire package as one serving, and thus undermine your attempt to control calories. You also need to be aware of ingredients you may not want added to your diet—at least not in the large amounts often put into energy bars. If the product is classified as a dietary supplement or the wrapper has a supplement facts panel printed on it, your energy bar will most likely contain larger amounts of vitamins, minerals, herbs, or caffeine, making your snack more of a drug than a food. For example, one of the energy bars I reviewed contained 50% of the RDA for iron. That's enough iron to pose serious health risks to men. Make sure you avoid energy bars that contain ephedra or ma huang, and guarana— herbs that can cause blood pressure problems, and in some instances, serious illness or death.

If you're looking for reputable, good-tasting energy bars, I suggest that you choose Kashi Go-lean, Luna, Met-Rx, and Genisoy—all of these brands contain a good amount of complex carbohydrates and fewer refined sugars.

# Which Fats First?

**Q:** *Why does my nutritionist tell me I need more essential fatty acids in my diet?*

**A:** Essential fatty acids (EFAs), like omega-3 and omega-6, are necessary components to our diet because every cell in the body must have them to survive. Our bodies can't make EFAs, so we have to eat foods that contain them. Omega-3 fatty acids can be found in flaxseeds and green leafy vegetables, and in high fat, coldwater fish like salmon, tuna, and mackerel. Omega-6 fatty acids are found in sesame and sunflower seeds as well as in evening primrose oil.

If you want to manage your weight, keep your heart strong, support your digestion, and boost your immunity, EFAs can help you. Essential fatty acids also support glandular and organ function, lubricate the joints, ease premenstrual syndrome (PMS), stimulate the production of fat-digesting enzymes, and help to keep you warm. Studies have shown that EFAs can effectively lower triglycerides, blood pressure, and risk of blood-clot formation. On the flip side, if you don't get enough EFAs, you may compromise your vision, learning ability and memory, energy level, and healing potential.

For you to receive the greatest benefit from the health-giving properties of EFAs, you need to eat them in the right ratio. Lipid experts suggest the ratio of omega-6 to omega-3 fatty acids should be about 2:1. This ratio isn't easily achieved because the American diet is far too high in omega-6 and dangerously low in omega-3 fats. Avoiding processed, hydrogenated fats and eating at least 15% of your daily calories from healthy fats can best achieve this favorable ratio. You can accomplish this by using unrefined olive and canola oils exclusively and taking flaxseed or fish oil supplements daily. Used in the right amounts and ratios, the right fats will provide invaluable health benefits.

Keep in mind that processing has damaged the majority of oils found on grocery store shelves; in addition, improper packaging and storage may have further degraded them. Choose only EFA-rich oils that have been pressed from organically grown seeds at low temperature under protection from light and oxygen, which destroy the essential oils. Once opened, you should consume bottled oils within a few months, so don't buy the bulk oils.

# Curative Cup of Brew?

**Q:** *What is Essiac tea and does it really stop tumors from growing?*

**A:** Essiac tea is an herbal mixture of burdock root, Indian rhubarb, sheep sorrel, and slippery elm bark. The tea is usually taken one to three times per day, on an empty stomach. It was formulated by an Ojibwa healer and given to cancer patients by a Canadian nurse (Rene Caisse—"Essiac" spelled backwards). Although this formula has been marketed as an immune booster, appetite stimulant, pain reliever, and tumor killer, there is no scientific evidence to support these claims. Most of the unpublished laboratory and clinical studies conducted by Caisse and her partner, Dr. Charles Brusch, contain incomplete data and may be biased.

After hearing testimonials from patients who had been treated with Essiac tea, the Canadian government approached Caisse for permission to analyze her formula. She refused. They eventually concluded that there was limited evidence to suggest that Essiac was effective as a cancer remedy, but did nothing to stop Caisse from continuing to use Essiac to treat patients.

It appears that Essiac tea is relatively safe to consume in the prescribed dosage and no adverse effects associated with the use of Essiac have been reported. Even if Essiac tea has been dismissed as a cancer cure, the research conducted on the individual herbs in this tea is worth mentioning. For example, a number of laboratory studies on burdock and Indian rhubarb indicate that both herbs contain high concentrations of anthraquinones, tannins, and polysaccharides that have been reported to provide cell protection and immune stimulation. In fact, a number of chemotherapies, including Adriamycin, are anthraquinone derivatives. Compounds similar to those found in slippery elm bark (fatty acids and fatty acid esters) also have demonstrated immune-boosting powers. Slippery elm bark has a high level of mucilage, which makes it very soothing for scratchy, raw sore throats. For this reason, I sometimes recommend Essiac tea to individuals who are undergoing radiation to the gastrointestinal tract.

You can find Essiac tea, manufactured by Essiac Products in New Brunswick, and another Canadian product—Flor-essence—believed to be an eight-herb recipe developed by Brusch and Caisse, widely available at health food stores.

# The Skinny on Fat Substitutes

**Q:** *Are fat substitutes safe to eat?*

**A:** According to a recent study by the Calorie Control Council, an association of low calorie and diet food manufacturers, nearly two-thirds of American adults consume low or reduced fat foods and beverages. Given the news that a high intake of fat is associated with increased risk of obesity, some types of cancer, and possibly gallbladder disease, I can see why health-conscious individuals are choosing foods made with fat substitutes in an attempt to improve their health or help them trim down.

Fat substitutes are meant to reduce a food's fat and calorie content while maintaining the texture provided by fat, but they often fall short on taste and versatility. In addition, one of the fat substitutes on the market today may lead to health problems.

Fat substitutes like Simplesse and Avicel (which are egg and milk protein-based fat substitutes) are used to create low fat versions of creamy yogurt, chips, cheese spreads and other snack foods. These food substitutes have been widely accepted as safe because they are digested and absorbed by the body in the same way that any food made with egg or milk would be. Unfortunately, you can't use them for cooking or baking because they can't withstand high temperatures like regular fats do.

Enter Olestra, a synthetic, indigestible fat substitute developed to be heat stable and to contribute no calories or fat to foods. Olestra is a chemical combination of sucrose (sugar) and fatty acids. Although Olestra was originally touted as a dieter's dream, early studies found that Olestra molecules were so large that they passed right through the intestinal tract and actually stained the underwear of test subjects! The manufacturers reformulated Olestra, but the nightmare appears to be continuing. Consumers have reported bloating, cramping, and diarrhea after eating as little as twenty Olestra-containing potato chips. Olestra also causes malabsorption of carotenoids, cell-protecting plant chemicals found in yellow, orange and red plants. A study reported in the *Journal of Clinical Nutrition* tested the effects of Olestra on consumers' blood levels of lycopene, a prostate-protecting carotenoid found in tomatoes. The study found that blood levels of lycopene in test subjects who ate just six potato chips per day for one month were 40% lower than in control subjects who didn't eat Olestra-containing foods.

It appears that removing fat from foods is not as easy as it sounds and we just don't know the long-term implications of consuming fat substitutes like Olestra. Although I wouldn't recommend eating substituted-fat products on a regular basis, I do think you could consume moderately sized portions of these products on occasion. More importantly, remember that some natural fats are good for your health. Not only do fats help us to absorb vitamins A, D, E and K, but they also are the only source of linoleic acid, an essential fatty acid that our bodies cannot manufacture and must get from food.

# Flax Facts

**Q:** *If I don't eat fish, should I consume flax?*

**A:** If you're looking for a way to get more omega-3 fatty acids into your diet, eating flaxseeds may be a perfect choice for you! Flaxseeds are rich in vitamins, minerals, and fiber and contain alpha linolenic acids, fats similar to those found in fish. Flaxseeds offer a wonderful array of health advantages!

Studies have shown that flaxseeds may lower total and LDL cholesterol levels, as well as blood pressure. Flaxseeds may also keep platelets from becoming sticky—potentially reducing chances of a heart attack. Flaxseeds have shown a lot of promise in preventing and fighting cancer, too. Population and experimental human studies have demonstrated that lignans, fiber compounds found in flax, can bind to estrogen receptors, inhibiting the onset of estrogen-stimulated breast cancer. Although some studies have indicated a diet high in alpha linolenic acids may increase the risk of prostate cancer, other studies show a reduction in risk when a low fat diet and lignan-rich flaxseeds are consumed. I believe that adding ground flaxseed to a diet supplemented with omega-3 and other essential fatty acids is the best course to take for optimal health.

It's pretty easy to include flaxseed in your diet because many food products contain flaxseed—look for flax in breads, cereals, and bakery goods. Bakers may use flaxseed flour or include flaxseed in baked goods. Flax is also used as a substitute for eggs in baked goods, although I haven't had great success with this—the products turn out very dense. I personally try to avoid heating flaxseed or oil in an effort to cash in on maximum omega-3 fatty acid benefits. I grind flaxseeds and sprinkle them over cold cereals and salads or in blenderized smoothies. Some people like the yellow color of golden flax, but it doesn't have any better nutritional profile than the more common brown flax. Flaxseed oil can be substituted for flax seeds, but I would caution you against taking flaxseed oil capsules, which contain very little omega-3 fatty acids!

When storing whole flaxseed, keep it in a clean, dry, airtight container at room temperature for up to a year. Once you grind flaxseed, there is greater risk of developing an off flavor and taste. That's why it's best to grind whole flaxseed as you need it. After grinding flaxseed, you should refrigerate any excess in an opaque container, but not for more than ninety days.

## Don't bite into those flax seeds just yet!

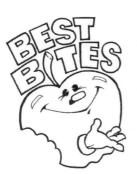

**Your teeth can't possibly chew through the tough exterior of the seeds to release the valuable oil within. Avoid the temptation of buying conveniently ground flaxseeds at the health food store, which may have been exposed to light, oxygen or heat.**

Use a hand-held coffee bean grinder and grind just what you need for your meal. Flaxseeds absorb about five times their volume of liquid, so make sure you drink plenty of purified water or juice every time you eat freshly ground flax.

# A Healthy Catch?

Q: *I want to eat more fish, but am afraid of mercury contamination. How can I avoid eating contaminated fish?*

A: The general rule of thumb is this: the larger the fish, the longer they've been swimming and feeding in contaminated waters, so they probably have accumulated more chemicals in their tissues. Mackerel and herring are examples of large, fatty fish that are most likely to contain dangerous chemicals like pesticides and heavy metals.

The pesticide DDT and industrial polychlorinated biphenyls (PCBs) are the chemicals of greatest concern. While these chemicals were outlawed in the U.S. in the 1970s, their residues still fill the ecosystem. And even if residues are in the decline, DDT used in other countries can eventually make its way into fish consumed in the U.S. Because mercury gas from industrial and household wastes is emitted into the air and water on a daily basis, nearly all fish have trace amounts of mercury in their systems. Fish near industrial regions are especially prone to increased mercury levels, which is why 40 states now issue regular advisories on mercury content in their freshwater fish. See www.epa.gov/waterscience/fish for a link to your state's advisory. Women of childbearing age and young children are advised to limit their consumption of fish and to avoid altogether species that may have high concentrations of chemicals.

Please don't misunderstand—despite the obvious health risks associated with eating fish, you should still eat about eight ounces of fish per week. Fish remain one of the healthiest low-calorie sources of protein, omega-3 fatty acids, and minerals. Fish with bones, such as canned salmon and sardines, are great nondairy sources of calcium. Eating fish has also been linked to reduced heart disease and lower cancer risk. For example, studies have shown that eating seafood at least twice a week can protect against heart attacks. At Johns Hopkins University, researchers discovered that even though mercury in fish may in fact raise the risk for heart disease, the omega-3 fatty acids from the fish seemed to undo mercury's detrimental effect, thereby reducing the overall risk of a heart attack. Studies have also confirmed that omega-3 fatty acids also may act to decrease inflammation, support immunity during radiation treatments, and reduce the risk of metastasis in a number of cancers.

It comes down to choosing fish wisely. The Food and Drug Administration suggests that shark, swordfish, king mackerel, and tilefish (known as golden snapper or golden bass) are not safe in any amount for at-risk individuals. Moderate mercury levels exist in tuna steaks, red snapper, American lobster, saltwater bass, halibut, and grouper, so consume these fish no more than once a month. The fish with the least mercury, according to the nonprofit Environmental Working Group, include blue crab, farmed catfish, flounder, haddock, salmon (farmed or wild), and shrimp. Also interesting to note: white albacore tuna, which is a larger, predatory fish, has about twice the mercury of light tuna.

# Fish Oil or Snake Oil?

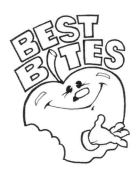

**One alternative to eating fish is to get omega-3 fatty acids from supplement pills containing oil from deep sea fish.**

The better the supplement quality, the less likely it will cause side effects like belching and nausea. And, the more likely you'll get what you paid for. An independent supplement review conducted by ConsumerLab.com found that some fish oil supplements didn't contain the claimed levels of the omega-3 fatty acids (EPA and DHA), and fell short by up to 67% of the levels of omega-3 fatty acids promised. When you purchase your fish oil supplements, make sure that they have been independently tested to be free of mercury, PCBs, and other contaminants. Most reputable manufacturers of fish oil and other supplements will provide these testing results if you just ask!

# Orange You Glad You Did?

**Q:** *I know I should eat more fruits and vegetables, but I really don't care for them. How can I get myself to eat more produce?*

**A:** Eating more fruits and vegetables isn't difficult, but it does take a degree of commitment and creativity. I ask people all the time if they like broccoli and sometimes I get a resounding, "No!" Then I find out that they've never tried broccoli! If you "think" that you don't like a certain fruit or vegetable, it's time to expand your horizons. Make an effort to eat at least one new plant food every month. You may find several new fruits or vegetables that you actually enjoy! Now the creative part—add finely chopped vegetables to egg omelets, soups, stews, and pasta sauces. You will hardly taste them! Raw veggies or fruit also make a great, low calorie snack while you're preparing dinner. And, if you blend frozen fruit with nonfat yogurt and juice, you can enjoy a healthful, refreshing fruit smoothie.

Too busy to peel, cut, chop, and cook fruit and vegetables? Eliminate preparation time by buying precut, ready-to-eat vegetables and prepared salads. Buy frozen vegetables and pop them into the microwave (preferably in a nonplastic container) to give yourself an additional serving or two of vegetables at dinnertime. When you're in a crunch for time, use canned and frozen fruit, bottled juices, and dried fruits. Raisins, dates, grapes, and cherry tomatoes can be eaten on the spot. Or, on days when you just can't seem to get in your produce quota, try adding a greens food, or concentrated whole foods, dietary supplement, like Juice Plus+.

If I can't appeal to your sense of adventure or need for speed, then think about this: eat produce for the health of it! It can be nearly impossible to lose weight and keep it off if you don't eat fruits and vegetables. Produce is a tasty, low calorie "filler" or replacement for higher calorie foods. Most people can go only so long on reduced portion sizes before they revert back to their old eating habits and regain their weight and then some. Scientists know that eating produce offers protection against diseases like heart disease, cancer and obesity. Produce offers you no fat, little sodium, lots of fiber and generous amounts of health-promoting antioxidants.

All of these health benefits and preparation tricks should justify a true-blue effort on your part to eat more produce. Work toward a goal of at least five servings (more is ideal!) of fruits and vegetables per day. Choose brightly colored produce. Generally, the darker the plant, the greater the health potential. For example, one serving of romaine lettuce contains almost eight times as much vitamin A as a serving of iceberg lettuce. And, including fresh fruits and vegetables in your diet will also provide you with enzymes that support digestion.

# What's the Big Stink?

**Q:** *Why is garlic so healthy and how much do I need?*

**A:** I once read that garlic is so good, it cures everything but ugly. After looking at all of the research conducted on garlic, I can see why garlic ranks as a superior herb, despite its stinky reputation.

Sulfur-containing plant chemicals (allicin, diallyl disulfide, and others) found in garlic have a number of health-promoting effects. These chemicals block toxins produced by bacteria and viruses, destroy the ability of germs to grow and reproduce, and may even help combat viruses—something no man-made drug is able to do. Garlic has also been shown to be helpful in the treatment of *Candida albicans*, an annoying and sometimes painful yeast infection.

Garlic offers cardiac protection too. It can decrease blood cholesterol levels and possibly raise HDL ("good" cholesterol). Garlic thins the blood, allowing it to more easily pass through vessels, thus reducing the risk for heart attack, stroke, and high blood pressure. There is even evidence to suggest that garlic can diminish fats already deposited in hardened arteries!

Cancer appears to be inhibited by garlic, particularly cancers of the mouth, digestive tract, breast, liver, and skin. Sulfur compounds found in allium vegetables like garlic, onions, and leeks are known for preventing the development of abnormal cells and slowing the progression of already established cancer cells. Garlic also has immune stimulatory characteristics, strengthening the body's defense against cancer.

To reap the therapeutic effects of garlic, you need to consume the equivalent of one clove per day (I said clove, not entire bulb!). Simply chop and throw raw garlic right into salads, stews, and casseroles, or bake the whole bulb in an oven at 350°F for twenty minutes and use as bread spread. Studies have shown that if you microwave garlic, the anti-cancer effects are lost. However, letting the crushed raw garlic sit at room temperature for ten minutes before microwaving will preserve most of its anti-cancer effects. While garlic cloves might be more potent, capsules can also be just as effective. In commercial supplements, a daily dose of at least 10 milligrams of allicin or a total allicin potential of 4,000 micrograms is suggested. If you're concerned about garlicky breath or body odor, try deodorized garlic supplements—they are a socially acceptable and effective alternative.

Some people have reported stomach irritation with garlic consumption, but garlic is considered to be a very safe and tolerable herb. Garlic can also kill friendly gut bacteria, so make sure that you take probiotics like lactobacillus or eat yogurt on a regular basis to keep your intestinal tract healthy.

# Laboratory Lentils

Q: *Should I be concerned about genetically modified foods?*

A: Although the National Academy of Sciences (NAS) has issued a statement that "there is no evidence that unique hazards exist in the use of recombinant DNA or in the movement of genes between unrelated organisms," I don't think you should assume genetically engineered (GE) foods are safe.

Food crops currently produced through biotechnology include soybeans, corn, rapeseed (canola), potatoes, rice, squash, and tomatoes. By removing genes from one plant or animal and placing them into another, food technologists can change ordinary food crops and animals into "superior" forms that can better resist pests and disease, grow faster, or contain more nutrients. The advantages to raising genetically engineered crops include less crop damage from insect infestation, which in turn, leads to less use of dangerous chemical pesticides. New products being developed include smaller, seedless melons for use as single servings, sweeter peas, and rice with more protein. Consumers benefit by enhanced flavor and freshness and improvements in taste and healthful qualities. Soybeans, for example, have been modified to contain higher levels of omega-3 fatty acids, the fats that are protective against heart disease, rheumatoid arthritis and cancer.

As good as genetically engineered foods sound, some researchers feel that any benefits to genetic engineering are outweighed by some major health risks. Some suggest that transplanted genes may alter the expression levels of native genes, resulting in foods that are toxic, allergenic, or otherwise harmful. We also don't know if genetic engineering changes phytochemical content of plant foods, even though genetic engineered and conventional foods typically have the same vitamin, mineral, protein and major nutrient profiles. In a recent study, however, genetically engineered soybeans were found to have decreased levels of beneficial phytoestrogens (plant chemicals that may calm hot flashes and decrease risk of some cancers) when compared to conventional soybeans. In another study published in the medical journal *Lancet,* rats fed genetically engineered potatoes developed damage to their organs and immune systems. The use of biotechnology could also introduce allergens into foods where none existed before. When scientists transferred an allergen from Brazil nuts to soybean plants, the engineered soybeans contained more lectins, which act as antigens, increasing allergic responses in consumers. The natural environment also may be affected by genetic engineering—we might end up with more aggressive weeds, or see a reduction in pest-eating insects due to harm from eating those insects or fungus that feed on genetically modified plants.

Genetically engineered foods are rampant in our food supply. At least 95% of soy and 90% of corn has been genetically altered and is used to feed the animals modern society raises for food. Every food made from genetically engineered plants, like corn syrup, corn starch, soy protein, and soy sauce, also adds altered plants to our diet. While there is no labeling law to identify foods that have been genetically modified, to avoid these foods and eat more safely, choose organic produce as often as possible and look for "non-GMO" on the labels of soy foods.

# Going With the Grain

**Q:** *Do you have any tips on how to include more whole grains in my diet?*

**A:** If you're like most people, you probably eat a good variety of bagels, pasta, and rice, but still only consume the equivalent of one whole grain item a day—far less than the current recommendation to eat at least three servings of whole grain foods each day.

The news has been out for quite a while now: eat more fiber rich whole grains and enjoy better health. Consuming bran from whole grains reduces blood levels of LDL, ("bad" cholesterol), promotes healthy detoxification, regulates blood sugar, and prevents constipation and more serious bowel problems like diverticulitis and colon polyps. Lignans found in whole grains may also reduce the risk of breast and prostate cancer. Harvard University investigators found that physicians who consumed whole grain cereal every day lowered their risk of dying over the next several years from any kind of disease by 17%, while those who ate refined cereals, on the other hand, had no such protection! Why are whole grains so much better than their refined forms? Whole grains contribute vitamin E, magnesium, selenium, and zinc— nutrients that are lost forever during the refinement process and not added back when refined foods are enriched.

Adding whole grains to your diet can be tricky business. "Rolled oats," "multi-grain," and "hearty wheat" are descriptors placed on food labels to help sell products to unsuspecting health-oriented consumers. I suggest that you ignore the fancy names on the front of the package and look on the back (or side) at the ingredients listing. The first ingredient must be "whole wheat" or "whole grain" for the product to qualify as a whole grain food.

Instant oatmeal, instant brown rice, and vegetable pastas are three notorious grain products that make you think you're eating healthier because they imply whole grain goodness.

The easiest way to include more whole grains in your diet is to start your day with a hearty, high fiber breakfast cereal. Try All Bran, Bran Buds, Kashi for Good Friends, or Raisin Bran. All of these brands deliver at least six or more grams of fiber per serving. As you make your way down the bread aisle, remember that brown isn't necessarily better. Some manufacturers add caramel coloring or molasses to their breads to give them a deep brown color. The Nutrition Facts panel can help you decide which breads are best—look for a product that provides at least 3 grams of dietary fiber per serving. Finally, grab a high fiber snack like air-popped popcorn, whole grain crackers, or fruit and bran muffins. Combine all of these whole grain choices with a variety of fruits, vegetables, and legumes and you'll be well on your way to getting the recommended 25 – 35 grams of dietary fiber per day.

For those of you who experience discomfort after eating high fiber foods, don't give up. A group of researchers at the University of California found that over time, the bacteria in your digestive tract adapt to accommodate the increase in fiber and produce less gas. You can help to minimize gas and bloating by increasing your fiber intake slowly. Add an additional serving or two of fruits or vegetables, a few slices of whole grain bread, or ½ cup of beans each week. And don't forget to drink more fluid too. Fiber holds water, making stools softer and easier to pass.

# Tea Time!

**Q:** *How much green tea do I need to drink every day in order to stay healthy?*

**A:** Anywhere between two and four cups per day is suggested to obtain health benefits. A study published in the American Heart Association journal *Circulation* found that almost 2,000 heart attack patients who drank at least two cups of tea every day had a 44% lower death rate than those who didn't drink tea at all. Green tea has a wonderfully unique flavor, but it's the health benefits that have consumers all abuzz. Studies have shown that green tea can fight bacterial and viral infections and may protect against a number of diseases. Tea's curative powers are most likely due to its antioxidant content—both black and green teas contain polyphenols, or catechins, plant chemicals that protect against cell-destroying free radicals.

Green tea is now accepted as a cancer preventative on the basis of numerous test tube, animal, and human population studies. Green tea works to prevent oxidation, inhibit the growth of cancer cells, and may possibly destroy cancer cells while maintaining the integrity of surrounding healthy cells. Researchers have also found that tea, with or without milk, may actually help strengthen bones in post-menopausal women. According to a study in the *American Journal of Clinical Nutrition,* women age sixty-five to seventy-five who drank at least one cup of tea every day had significantly higher bone density than women who didn't drink tea. Tea's good for the heart too. A different study concluded that women who consumed one or more cups of tea per day were 54% less likely to have hardening of the arteries—a condition that can lead to heart attack and stroke. Another study, conducted at Harvard Medical School, found that heart attack patients who drank at least two cups of tea every day were 44% less likely to die than those who didn't drink tea.

Before you put the kettle on, remember that tea contains caffeine, which can cause nervousness, sleeplessness, and heart rate irregularities in some individuals. Tea also contains nutrients that can bind to calcium and other minerals, so you shouldn't consume tea at the same time you take mineral supplements.

# The Latest Buzz

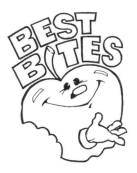

**If you're trying to limit your caffeine intake, you might want to think before you switch to decaf.**

According to a variety of tea company representatives and the London Tea Council, solvents used to decaffeinate tea can decrease the amount of health-promoting chemicals by up to 60%. It might be more practical to drink a cup or two of regular green tea during the early part of the day and consume other foods high in beneficial polyphenols, like red grapes, kidney beans, raisins, prunes, or an occasional glass of red wine.

## How powerful is your tea?

| Tea | Catechins |
| --- | --- |
| Green tea | 27% |
| Oolong tea | 23% |
| Black tea | 4% |
| Herbal tea | 0% |

# Greener Pastures

**Q:** *Should I take a greens supplement?*

**A:** I believe that our highly processed diet doesn't give us all the essential vitamins, minerals, and enzymes that we need for proper functioning. And even if we eat plenty of broccoli, it's probably still a good idea to explore the world of green superfoods (alfalfa, barley grass, wheatgrass) and algaes (chlorella and spiriluna). These greens are some of the most nutritious of all plant foods—high in amino acids, proteins, fiber, enzymes, and packed with antioxidants like carotenoids and chlorophyll. Greens are sold in extract and liquid form and are marketed to consumers wishing to improve digestion, increase energy, and cleanse the body. Choosing the right kind of green food depends on your overall health goals. Keep in mind that if you are on blood-thinning medications, you should take greens supplements on a consistent basis. Here's a brief glimpse of the best and brightest:

Alfalfa sprouts contain saponins, a plant chemical that has been shown to lower fat and reduce LDL ("bad" cholesterol). Saponins also play a valuable role in preventing hardening of the arteries and stimulating the immune system by increasing the activity of natural killer cells, such as T-lymphocytes and interferon. Although sprouts of any kind are highly nutritious, many should be consumed with caution because they are linked to an increased incidence of food-borne illnesses.

Wheat and barley grasses are particularly good sources of calcium, iron and B vitamins. As one of the best sources of quality chlorophyll, these grasses may be potent blood purifiers and liver detoxifiers. You can gulp down freshly squeezed grasses from a health food store or purchase them as a dried powder.

Spirulina, a blue-green algae, may play a role in fighting cancer. A number of studies have shown that spirulina and chlorella extracts significantly increase natural killer cell activity and may protect against the harmful effects of chemotherapy and radiation. Choose only spirulina that has been tested for heavy metals and cyanotoxins (toxins that may have been inadvertently harvested along with the spirulina).

# Out of the Frying Pan and into the Grill

**Q:** *Is it healthy to eat grilled meats?*

**A:** Before you stoke up the coals (or turn on the gas), you should know that grilled meats could be hazardous to your health. High-heat methods of cooking, like frying, barbecuing, and grilling, can cause meat, chicken, and fish to produce compounds called heterocyclic amines (HCAs). Heterocyclic amines are known to be carcinogenic (cancer-causing). To add fuel to the proverbial flame, when fats from grilled meats drip onto the hot coals, other carcinogens, called polycyclic aromatic hydrocarbons (PAHs), are produced. These PAHs migrate back onto the grilled foods when smoke or flames blacken, or char, the meat.

Population studies show a strong link between people who eat grilled meats regularly and the increased incidence of stomach, colorectal, and breast cancer. In fact, a University of Minnesota study found that women who consumed just three well-done meats per week increased their risk of breast cancer by 462%!

With that kind of news you might be tempted to say goodbye to your barbecue. No need for that, though, as long as you take steps to reduce the health risks when you grill. First, choose lean cuts of meats like beef or pork, skinless chicken, and fish. The less fat in the meat, the less PAHs are formed. Next, marinate your meats with citrus juice, vinegar-based marinades, or olive oil before grilling. These ingredients contain natural plant chemicals and vitamins that can significantly reduce the production of HCAs.

You can also reduce exposure to carcinogens if you cut grilling time by partially steaming, boiling, or microwaving your meat before grilling. Don't pierce meat with a fork while grilling because juice from the meat will escape and drip onto the coals. Instead, use tongs or a spatula to turn the meat. If you intend to baste your meat with a barbecue or teriyaki glaze, wait until the meat is almost done. Sauces tend to cause flare-ups. Finally, don't eat burnt or charred meats. Try grilling a medley of vegetables like squash, zucchini, peppers, and onions for a flavorful, healthy side dish. Or, toss this colorful mixture over some beans and brown rice and enjoy a savory and satisfying plant-based meal. Most importantly, remember that eating grilled foods once in a while is not a concern. It's the long-term and frequent exposure to these grilling compounds that increases your cancer risk.

## Healthy grilling basics for every backyard chef:

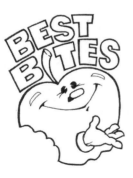

- Clean the grill before you cook
- Precook meats by baking, broiling or microwaving
- Cook over a low heat to avoid flare-ups
- Choose low fat meats like chicken breast or lean beef
- Flip frequently
- Remove charred and burned portions before eating

# Natural Immune Power!

**Q:** *I can't seem to shake off my cold; are there foods that I can eat to help me boost my immune system?*

**A:** If you're sick of being sick, you'll be relieved to know that you can boost your body's natural healing abilities by changing your diet. The first step is to make sure you're consuming enough calories and protein—without the appropriate amounts of fuel and building blocks, you won't produce healthy new cells (including cells of the immune system). Weight loss has a negative impact on immunity, so if you're underweight, you'll need additional calories to help you regain some weight. Ask a dietitian to determine your calorie and protein needs and advise you about "healthy" high-calorie foods.

Now, let's take a serious look at what you're eating—if it's fried foods, foods made with hydrogenated oils like margarines and shortening, or lots of polyunsaturated vegetable oils (corn, safflower, soybean, and others), you could be suppressing your immune system. Make sure you choose fats rich in monounsaturated fatty acids (olive and canola) and omega-3 fatty acids (cold water fish and flax). These fats not only benefit the heart, they also support immunity.

A diet of highly refined carbohydrates can wreak havoc on the immune system as well, so decrease your intake of high sugar junk foods and get your sweet fix from the natural sugars found in fruits. To increase your antioxidant levels, eat plenty of colorful fruits and vegetables, which are rich in flavonoids. Garlic, green tea, and certain edible mushrooms (maitake, shiitake, and enoki) also have proven immune-enhancing effects.

Consider taking a daily antioxidant dietary supplement containing carotenoids, vitamins C and E, and selenium. These powerhouse nutrients can limit the amount of damage done by free radicals; they also support immunity by stimulating the production of lymphocytes, which assist in the neutralization of toxic molecules, and enhancing macrophage and T-killer cell activity. Echinacea and astragalus are two herbs that have demonstrated antiviral and immune-boosting effects. Taken at the first sign of a cold, these herbs may reduce the severity and duration of your illness.

Finally, take a serious look at your current lifestyle. If you stop smoking, get enough sleep and exercise, follow safe food handling procedures in the kitchen, and reduce your stress, you can support your body's healing processes naturally!

# Pumping up Iron

**Q:** *I'm slightly anemic but I don't want to take constipating iron supplements. What kinds of foods contain the most iron?*

**A:** Liver, meat, fish, and poultry are the best sources of iron because they contain heme iron, which is most easily absorbed by the body. Some plants, like iron-enriched grains, green leafy vegetables, and potatoes contain a good amount of iron, but the iron tends to be poorly absorbed by your body when you eat these foods.

Although I wouldn't "beef" up on animal foods, to boost your absorption of iron from vegetable sources, you might try adding just a few chunks of meat to a vegetarian dish. Also, because vitamin C promotes iron absorption, add more vitamin C-rich foods like citrus fruits or juice, broccoli, cabbage, and tomatoes to your iron-boosting diet.

Preparing your meals in cast iron cookware (the iron leaches into the food when heated) also will increase the iron content of your meals. Although spinach, kale, beets, and Swiss chard are good sources of iron, they contain oxalic acid, which reduces iron absorption. So, you may want to limit servings of these foods. Calcium-rich dairy foods and tea and coffee also interfere with iron absorption, so try to limit dairy intake to one serving per day and drink water in place of these beverages. I would also avoid over-the-counter antacids like Tums—iron is poorly absorbed in a low acid environment.

Once you increase your iron intake, it usually takes at least six months to improve you blood count and replenish your body's iron stores, so be patient. If your dietary efforts aren't successful, consider supplementation. Before you run to the drugstore for some iron, you need to know that anemia has a number of causes, including vitamin B12 or folate deficiency. Your doctor can run routine blood tests— serum iron, TIBC, and ferritin—to determine if you are truly iron deficient. I urge you to take this additional step, because if you take iron and don't need it, you may increase your risk of heart disease, diabetes, and cancer (iron can be a pro-oxidant and cause cell destruction!).

If you find out that you are low in iron, consider using dessicated liver as a high quality, concentrated form of iron. It's available in powder, pill, and liquid form and contains B vitamins and copper—nutrients essential for rebuilding red blood cells. I recommend a liquid extract derived from organically grown beef.

The most common side effects of iron supplementation include constipation, cramping, and stomach upset. To reduce these unpleasant side effects, you need to either increase your absorption of iron from your iron supplement, by taking some vitamin C, or by starting with half the recommended dose of iron at mealtimes. For even better iron absorption, avoid taking iron with vitamin E or zinc. Drinking plenty of fluid, maintaining a high fiber diet, eating flax seeds and taking a natural vegetable laxative such as Senokot can help promote elimination.

# Rejuvenating Juice

Q: *Can I gain more energy and boost my immune system if I begin a juicing program?*

A: Thousands of people are slurping down pineapple-blueberry-banana or watercress-kale-carrot concoctions in an effort to feel energized, fight disease, strengthen immunity, or just find an easy way to get the recommended amount of produce into their diet. With our fast-paced lifestyles, I can't blame them. After all, most of us are lucky if we eat two servings of the suggested nine servings of produce each day! If you approach juicing with some common sense, it can be a valuable component of a balanced diet and help you achieve your health goals.

Ideal candidates for juicing therapy include individuals who are no longer in cancer treatment, those who are not losing weight, or those who are strong and just want to flush out their systems. I would suggest investing in a rotary blade juicer; these juicers are very good at extracting juice and are moderately priced. If you plan on juicing several times a day, get a juicer with a compressor. Sometimes, the juicer manufacture includes a pamphlet of juice recipes; if not, you can get suggestions from any number of juicing books available at bookstores. Use organic produce as often as possible. Plants grown without pesticides and herbicides tend to contain higher levels of nutrients and pose less of a health threat than regular produce. To support immunity by keeping blood sugar levels in check, it's important to drink your juice with a protein-based meal or snack.

If you're in the middle of chemotherapy or radiation treatments, adding fresh juice to a whole foods diet may assist in detoxification, but drinking large amounts of juice or fasting on juice is not recommended during this time. Sometimes, a one- or two-day juicing regimen can be followed during the early stages of cancer treatment or as a preventative to recurrence. Talk to a nutritionist if you want to follow a juicing program.

If you're immunocompromised, and your absolute neutrophil count (ANC) is low, you'll need to avoid all raw produce to reduce your risk of bacterial infection. Wait for the green light from your doctor before consuming freshly squeezed juices or other raw plant foods.

Individuals who have difficulty controlling their blood sugar need to be especially careful about drinking larger amounts of juice. Fresh juices require minimal digestion, so natural sugars from fruits and vegetables are released quickly into the bloodstream, rapidly raising blood sugar levels. Although fruits tend to contain the most sugar, beets and carrots can also cause a sharp rise in blood sugar. Adding soy or whey protein powder to your juices can help slow the release of sugars into the bloodstream.

If you're in a weakened state, have lost weight, or are recovering from surgery, juicing is not indicated. Remember that juices are very low in calories and protein. To support rebuilding, you should focus on foods and beverages that will provide you with adequate levels of calories and nutrients.

# A "Senior" Moment?

**Q:** *As a middle-aged woman (forty-something), I find that my memory is not what it used to be. What types of foods and/or supplements can I take to help improve my memory?*

**A:** Not only is losing your memory frustrating, it's probably causing you a bit of anxiety—after all, most people who feel their memory is fading tend to think "Alzheimers." Although memory loss is a common disorder in the elderly, most memory lapses in middle age have more to do with other consequences of aging—insufficient blood supply to the brain, free radical damage to brain tissue, hormonal imbalances (you may be perimenopausal), or excessive psychosocial stress. Raising adolescent children, caring for aged parents, working long hours, or experiencing a life-changing event like moving or getting a divorce can take an emotional, mental, and physical toll, especially on a woman who continually supports others while neglecting her own health (you know who you are!).

Changing your eating habits, along with exercise and relaxation, should help you deal with stress more positively. Don't skip meals or indulge in too much fat or sugar. Eat whole foods and plenty of fruits and vegetables chock full of anti-aging, cell-protecting chemicals. Limit processed and refined foods like sugar, white rice, and breads. Researchers at New York University School of Medicine concluded that individuals with high levels of sugar in the blood did worse on short-term memory tests. Simple sugars also deplete the body of many nutrients, particularly the B vitamins, which support the nervous system and our ability to adapt to stress. Consider adding to your diet an assortment of soy foods like soy milk or tofu that contain plant estrogens that may help balance fluctuating estrogen levels.

Besides a multivitamin (what...did you forget to take that, too?) you may want to take a B-complex 100 and either evening primrose oil or coldwater-fish-oil capsules. These dietary supplements can support mental clarity by improving circulation and nervous system function. If you're thinking about reaching for the gingko biloba, you should know that researchers don't agree on whether or not gingko helps to reverse memory loss. They do accept, however, that gingko contains powerful antioxidants that may protect the brain from oxidative damage.

# It is said that the best advice is free.

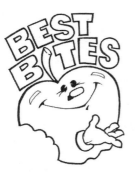

**If you want to improve your memory, just breathe deeply.**

Oxygen helps "feed" the brain, increasing your mental alertness— and it won't cost you a thing!

# A Daily Dose of Health

**Q:** *Do I need a multivitamin?*

**A:** The debate over whether or not most of us need a multivitamin may never end, but the idea has finally received serious consideration from mainstream medicine. The American Medical Association appears to have recognized that it is theoretically impossible to consistently eat a quality diet and that, for a variety of reasons, it is extremely unlikely that a typical person will consume the recommended amounts of every nutrient every day. In two landmark articles published in the June 2002 issue of the *Journal of the American Medical Association*, researchers suggested that all adults should probably take a vitamin and mineral supplement to help prevent chronic diseases, especially if their diets are substandard.

The need for dietary supplementation is not new to nutritionists. Today's fast-paced lifestyle lends itself to prepackaged, quickly cooked foods that have been stripped of life-sustaining nutrients; we simply don't take the time to eat and cook right. Population studies show that as many as 80% of Americans don't consume enough of the recommended dietary allowances for several nutrients, increasing their risk for subclinical nutrient deficiency. Because these deficiencies are marginal, signs and symptoms of clinical depletion may not be apparent; however, people still experience fatigue, lack of mental sharpness, or restlessness that can't be explained.

People who are at risk for poor nutrient status include weight watchers who are on any kind of restrictive diet; individuals who take prescription drugs, smoke tobacco, and overindulge in alcohol, caffeine, or fatty foods; those who avoid exercise; and people who are plagued with digestive disorders or chronic medical conditions. Even if you don't fit into any of these categories and think you eat right, you still might need to supplement your diet. A recent survey conducted by the United States Department of Agriculture revealed that 40% of people were "dietary optimists," reporting that their diets were excellent or good, when in fact, they weren't!

The benefits of taking vitamins, minerals, and accessory nutrients are numerous: they protect cells, support tissues and organs, and help enzymes complete chemical reactions in your body. Without these chemical reactions, you wouldn't be able to tie your shoes, read this book, or remember the question you just asked. Without adequate nutrition, the body begins to change biochemically, eventually leading to poor organ function, low energy utilization, and a dysfunctional immune system.

It's important to remember that dietary supplements don't replace a healthy diet. You'll get limited benefit from taking a one-a-day vitamin in an effort to counteract the damaging effects of that cheeseburger you just washed down with a diet cola. Scientists have recognized that nature has conveniently wrapped up vitamins, minerals, fiber, and special plant chemicals into wholesome food packages that are far superior to those found in supplements, so it just makes sense to eat right as a first priority and take vitamins as a secondary nutritional approach to health.

# Some supplemental advice:

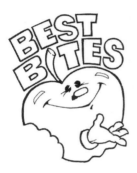

**Don't worry if you skip your daily dose of vitamins now and then. Most vitamins and minerals stay in the body and continue to work for a few days.**

Take your daily multivitamin with a citrus juice (orange, grapefruit or tomato). The acids in the fruits help to break down the supplements and may speed up their absorption.

If you have trouble swallowing supplements, try taking them with thickened liquids, like fruit nectars, or choose supplements that come in chewable or liquid form.

Avoid allergic reactions to dietary supplements by buying brands that don't contain fillers, additives or coal tars. Products that are additive-free proudly claim it on the label.

*For maximum absorption of nutrients, always divide your doses over the course of the day.*

# Mushrooms as Medicine

**Q:** *Do mushrooms have any health benefits?*

**A:** Mushrooms are more than a delicious addition to a salad or casserole; they contain protein, fiber, B vitamins, vitamin C, and calcium, as well as some unique compounds offering a number of substantial health benefits.

Of the roughly 38,000 species of mushrooms known, three kinds have demonstrated phenomenal healing potential: maitake, shiitake, and reishi. These medicinal mushrooms may lower the risk of cancer, boost immunity, protect the heart, ward off viral and bacterial infections, reduce inflammation, combat allergies, and support the body's ability to detoxify.

Doctors in Japan have long used maitake to lower blood pressure and blood lipids, two key risk factors in cardiovascular disease. Animal studies have shown that a particular molecule called X-fraction found in maitake may reduce insulin resistance, potentially helping people with non-insulin-dependent diabetes mellitus (NIDDM).

Maitake has also demonstrated effectiveness against leukemia, and stomach and bone cancers. In fact, some studies found that cancer patients who took maitake experienced relief from chemotherapy side effects like loss of appetite, vomiting, nausea, and low white blood cell counts. You can find maitake d-fraction in powdered extracts and liquid tinctures.

Shiitake mushrooms may help the body combat heart disease, cancer, and viruses.

One Japanese study identified a specific amino acid in shiitake that helps speed up the processing of cholesterol in the liver. Like maitake, shiitake also appears to fight cancer.

A polysaccharide called lentinan, isolated from shiitake, has been found to cause tumors to shrink in animal studies. Shiitake mushrooms have a very appealing flavor and are sometimes used as an alternative to meat. Shiitake and rice bran capsules are often sold in health food stores.

Through test tube and human studies, reishi has demonstrated antiallergenic, anti-inflammatory, antiviral, antibacterial, and antioxidant properties. Laboratory tests also indicate that reishi may help fight tumors and may help individuals with asthma and other respiratory complaints. Reishi is reportedly used as a mood elevating substance, although I could find no clinical research to back up that claim. Reishi is available in tinctures, tablets, and by injection.

# Washing Away the Danger

**Q:** *Should I buy organic?*

**A:** If you want to lower your intake of synthetic herbicides and fungicides, or if you're concerned about the hormones found in the fatty portion of meats, eggs, and dairy foods, buying organic seems like the right thing to do. I've seen limited research concluding that some organic produce contains higher levels of nutrients than conventionally grown produce—but that doesn't necessarily mean that all foods labeled "organic" are healthful or nutritious. If you prefer the taste of and can afford organic products, you have plenty of choices. According to the nonprofit organization Organic Alliance, sales of organic products have grown by over 20% each year since 1990. In an effort to meet consumer demand, supermarkets are adding more and more organic products to their shelves.

No matter what kinds of organic foods you buy, read labels carefully. To be labeled "certified organic," which is the highest organic standard set by the USDA, foods must be grown, handled, and processed in compliance with organic standards. Farmers and processors must have detailed paperwork of their practices, and use of synthetic pesticides and fertilizers, genetic engineering, and irradiation are forbidden. Other labels may sound healthy, but are misleading. For example, animal products are "Raised Without Antibiotics" but aren't double-checked by the government to ensure claim accuracy. To meet the requirement for labeling chicken "Free Range," a farm need only keep chicken coop doors open a mere five minutes per day. The term "Natural" is a vague descriptor for products that have been minimally processed and contain no artificial ingredients or colors.

If you choose not to buy organic products, you can reduce the amount of pesticides you consume by washing and scrubbing fresh fruits and vegetables under running water with a sturdy vegetable brush. Surfactant cleaners like Basic H, Veggie Wash, and Organiclean help to remove dirt and pesticides that reside in nooks and crannies of plants like lettuce, broccoli, and herbs. It's also helpful to select produce without cuts, insect holes, mold, or decay, and to discard outer leaves of leafy vegetables. You can reduce stored residues of some pesticides by trimming fat from meat and poultry. Finally, select a variety of foods to reduce your exposure to a single type of pesticide or contaminant.

## Safest picks for organic news:

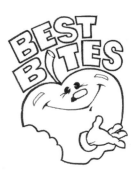

**www.allorganiclinks.com**
(Links to companies offering organic goods and services)

**www.ota.com**
(Organic Trade Association)

**www.panna.org**
(Pesticide Action Network)

**www.ewg.org**
(Shopping guide to pesticides in produce)

# Plastics: A Bad Wrap?

**Q:** *Is it safe to use plastic wrap when cooking or reheating foods in the microwave?*

**A:** Just when making dinner got easier, along comes a possible health risk associated with reheating leftovers in the microwave! Studies have shown that plasticizers, the compounds that give some plastic wraps their pliability, are suspected of causing cancer. Even small amounts of these compounds have caused genetic damage in animals. Other plasticizers, like DEHA (found in some plastic wraps) and bisphenol-A (found in the lining of metal cans and some baby bottles), may be potential hormone disrupters. Other research suggests that chemicals from plastics may migrate into your food—whether it is heated or not. For example, foods left in take-out containers for a period of time actually developed a plastic taste, and microwaved foods that touched plastic wrap were found to have transferred plastic at the point of contact. For these reasons, I suggest that you limit your exposure to certain plastics.

While we can't avoid all plastics, there are some easy things you can do to limit your exposure to unwanted chemicals. Begin by choosing containers that will least likely react with your foods. Plastic storage containers that are meant to take your food from "freezer to microwave" can break down with repeated heating and cooling and plastic compounds may migrate into your food. To be safe, I'd transfer frozen foods from plastic storage containers to a Pyrex or Corningware glass container before heating. Generally, the more rigid the plastic, the less likely the plastic compounds will transfer when heated, but I recommend using Tupperware and CrystalWare for storage only. When choosing a storage container, remember that fatty foods and highly acidic foods tend to absorb more plasticizers than other foods, so use a very rigid plastic container for these kinds of foods. Try to keep plastic wrap from touching any part of the foods that you heat and avoid heating foods in containers like margarine tubs or plastic containers that are not labeled microwave safe.

# The Good Bugs

**Q:** *What are probiotics?*

**A:** Anything—drinks, yogurts, dietary supplements—that contains "friendly" bacteria is considered to be a probiotic. Mounting research indicates that specific strains of bacteria, particularly *Lactobacillus GG, Lactobacillus johnsoni,* and *Bifidobacterium,* can alleviate diarrhea, lactose intolerance, inflammatory bowel disease, and other digestion-related maladies. There is also preliminary evidence that probiotics may have some cancer-fighting and immune-stimulating effects. A new study from Switzerland found that probiotics might actually help reduce populations of harmful bacteria in the nose, reducing risk for illnesses like pneumonia and strep throat.

The digestive tract is home to more than 400 species of bacteria, which can be depleted if we use antibiotics, are under stress, or eat a diet of highly processed, low-fiber foods. Probiotic therapy, using cultured foods or dietary supplements containing live bacteria, helps to replenish normal bacterial flora of the colon and prevent overgrowth of disease-producing bacteria.

In a typical grocery store, you can find a variety of buttermilk, kefir, and yogurt products—from kefir drinks to squeezable and drinkable yogurt. I recommend choosing low fat kefir products; plain, nonfat yogurt; or cultured soy yogurt if you're concerned about limiting your sugar and saturated fat intake. And yes, some bacteria can survive freezing, so frozen yogurt can be a nice, gut-enhancing treat once in a while.

If you consume three cups of yogurt per week, you should be able to maintain a healthy count of intestinal bacterial. If you have active disease or have just finished taking antibiotics, you may want to eat a cup of yogurt daily or take probiotic dietary supplements. Typical doses of probiotics range from one to ten billion colony-forming units (CFU) a few times per week. Always check labels of dietary supplement packages to ensure that the product has not expired; otherwise, you may end up purchasing inactive bacteria.

Most probiotic supplements are well tolerated, but if you do experience gas or constipation with use, consider adding a prebiotic (a nondigestible food containing ingredients like oligosaccharides and inulins), which may enhance the effectiveness of probiotics.

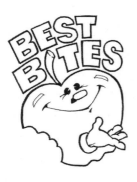

## Go Buggy!

**Yummy yogurt tubes from Stonyfield Farm, called Yosqueeze, are low in calories, fat, and sugar and give you the perfect excuse to try yogurt if you never have—they're fun to eat!**

If you'd rather slurp, Dannon makes a drinkable yogurt called Dannon Frusion Fruit n'Yogurt Smoothie. This delicious treat will cost you only about 270 calories and comes in a variety of palate-pleasing flavors.

# Protein Power!

**Q:** *How do I know if I'm getting enough protein in my diet?*

**A:** If you're a healthy individual, your diet should contain between 15 and 20% protein, which amounts to between 75 and 100 grams of protein if you eat 2,000 calories per day (protein provides four calories per gram). Getting enough protein doesn't seem to be a problem for most of us. Partly to blame are restaurants that serve 16-ounce steaks and double cheeseburgers—but then again, we choose to eat them now, don't we?

The good news is that once you know what your protein requirements are, you can confidently reorganize your meal composition to reduce animal-based foods and still get enough protein to maintain wellness. As you decrease the amount of animal proteins you consume, you should increase the amount of plant proteins on your plate. For example, a meal consisting of small bits of broccoli and rice surrounding a heap of meat should be replaced with a plate full of plants that may, or may not, be complemented by a small side portion of animal meat or dairy product.

If you eat a balanced, varied diet complete with lots of fruits and vegetables, legumes, raw nuts (walnuts, almonds, and pecans), seeds, soy (tempeh, seitan, tofu, edamame, soynuts), and limited amounts of animal flesh and dairy foods, you'll easily get enough protein to meet your body's needs. Building a high-protein, plant-based meal is easier than you think. Try adding nuts, seeds, and wheat germ to casseroles, breads, muffins, and cookies. Spread nut butters on sandwiches, toast, crackers or use as a dip for raw fruit slices. Cook and use dried peas, beans, and lentils in soups and pasta dishes.

If you decide to stop eating animal foods, make sure that you take a vitamin B12 dietary supplement. You may also need supplemental zinc and iron, as these nutrients are sometimes deficient in a vegetarian diet. If you want to forego dairy products, eat plenty of calcium-rich vegetables like collards, spinach, and broccoli, and choose calcium-fortified soy milk and orange juice.

# Ready to Go Raw?

**Q:** *Is it healthy to eat a diet of mostly raw foods?*

**A:** There are some practical and healthful reasons to eat a raw foods diet. You certainly won't have to cook as much and you'll spend less time reading food labels! In terms of nutritional impact, uncooked plants are high in a number of nutrients and retain their enzyme activity, which is important because enzymes assist in the digestion and absorption of food. You can lose weight on a raw foods diet and you might be able to fight disease, too. Current research on laboratory animals shows that eating less food may slow aging and decreases the incidence of some types of cancer and autoimmune diseases. Eating raw foods helps to boost energy levels, promote detoxification, and increase resistance to colds and flu—all natural side effects of a restricted calorie intake.

The raw foods, or living foods, diet plan calls for at least 75% of meals to be uncooked and encourages you to choose fruits, vegetables, sprouts, nuts, seeds, grains, sea vegetables, and other organic and natural foods that haven't been processed. Raw food connoisseurs can make attractive, creative, and delicious meals by using food processors and dehydrators. These food preparation methods ensure that foods are never heated above 106 degrees, the temperature at which enzymes start to die. Raw food preparation books are available at major bookstores and can help you plan your meals.

Before you toss out your frying pan, you should know that not everyone can, or should, eat a diet consisting primarily of raw foods. If you have difficulty chewing or swallowing, or have special health concerns, then a diet based on raw foods might be frustrating and detrimental to your overall wellness. People with digestive tract disorders like diverticulitis or ulcerative colitis, or anyone undergoing chemotherapy or radiation, may suffer from gas, bloating, spasms, or erratic bowel habits if they consume too many raw vegetables, fruits, and nuts. Additionally, anyone who has a significantly depressed white blood cell count could increase their risk for bacterial infections if they consume uncooked foods. It also may be difficult to get enough dietary protein from a vegan, raw foods diet. A generous intake of fruits and vegetables, legumes, and sprouted seeds provides at most about 50 grams of protein daily—not enough for someone who needs to gain weight, repair cells, rebuild stamina, or recover from surgery.

I believe the healthiest nutrition plan is one that focuses on whole foods and encourages a variety of foods prepared in different ways. Not all nutrients are lost when foods are cooked. And some nutrients, like lycopenes and other carotenoids found in red and orange fruits and vegetables, are actually more easily absorbed by the body if the foods are cooked instead of consumed raw. I've also learned that the longer you cook corn, the more antioxidant activity it will have! If you like the idea of adding more raw foods to your diet, I suggest you increase the amount of fresh fruits or vegetables that you currently eat. Then, try to incorporate raw nuts and cooked legumes into meals and snacks. For most people, making these simple dietary changes will positively impact their health without drastically changing their lifestyle or eating habits.

# Sprout alert!

**Children, the elderly, pregnant, or immunocompromised individuals should avoid eating raw sprouts.**

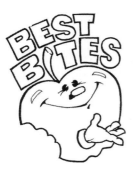

Alfalfa, clover, mung bean, and radish sprouts have been found to be contaminated with E.coli, the bacteria associated with serious illness and even death. The latest reports show that people who eat sprouts are five to ten times more likely to suffer from food poisoning than those who do not!

*If you're going to eat sprouts, always cook them, even when they are home grown. Harmful bacteria found in the seeds can multiply to illness-causing levels during sprouting. If you're concerned about losing valuable enzyme activity, stick to other raw plants like lettuce, carrots, and radishes. You can also eat raw broccoli, radish, and sunflower sprouts—they are free of natural toxins.*

# To Your Good Health?

Q: *Will drinking red wine lower my risk of a heart attack?*

A: People who drink one to two glasses of red wine each day may indeed have lower rates of heart disease and cancer. Chemicals in wine, called polyphenols, are powerful antioxidants that can reduce the rate and level at which our bodies suffer oxidative stress, which in turn kills cells and triggers diseases. Polyphenols can also be found in fruits, vegetables, tea, whole grains, and seeds.

Now, should you uncork the white wine or the red? As it turns out, scientists have confirmed that red wine offers more health benefits than white wine. A study from South America revealed that subjects who ate a high fat diet and who drank a glass of red wine each day reduced the amount of oxidative damage to their DNA by 50% and increased their levels of HDL (good cholesterol) by 14%. Conversely, those who consumed white wine lowered their DNA damage by 16% and increased their HDL by 9%. Wine is also a powerful cancer fighter. A test tube study published in the British medical journal, *BJU International*, concluded that components of red wine induced apotosis (self destruction) of human prostate cancer cells.

While studies show a definite beneficial link between alcohol and disease prevention, drinking too much can be risky. Studies have also shown that even one alcoholic drink per day may increase the risk of breast and esophageal cancer, and that higher levels of alcohol may increase your chances for coronary artery disease, liver disease, and hip fractures. Alcohol adds extra calories to your diet as well, making it harder to control your weight. Red wine also contains sulfites that can cause migraine headaches or allergic reactions in susceptible individuals.

If you want the cardiovascular and health-protecting effects of red wine without the alcohol, I suggest that you eat plenty of fruits and vegetables and drink purple grape juice. The U.S. Department of Agriculture states that purple grape juice contains more than three times the antioxidants contained in other juices! Researchers at Georgetown University found that people who drank about two cups of purple grape juice daily for two weeks produced a chemical that promotes widening of the blood vessels to the heart and serves as a powerful anticlotting agent. Now that's something to cheer about!

# Shark Cartilage: Another Fish Tale?

**Q:** *Does shark cartilage have any beneficial properties for cancer patients?*

**A:** Proponents suggest shark cartilage can reduce tumor size and slow or stop the growth of cancer, but shark cartilage proved worthless in a scientific study conducted by the Cancer Treatment Research Foundation in Arlington Heights, Illinois, and published in the *Journal of Clinical Oncology.* Researchers found that commercial-grade shark cartilage had no anticancer activity and no effect on the quality of life in cancer patients. As research has continued, however, scientists have discovered that there is a specific protein in cartilage that can block the formation of new blood vessels—a process called antiangiogenesis. The National Cancer Institute is currently conducting human trials using this cartilage derivative.

Beyond the need for more evidence, shark cartilage can be very costly (some patients reportedly spend over $500 per month) and overwhelming to consume. For example, a typical dosage of shark cartilage is 1 gram of shark cartilage for every kilogram of body weight. If you weigh 150 pounds (68 kg), you would need 68 grams of shark cartilage. To meet this requirement, you would have to consume 90 capsules (750 mg each) daily. If you decide to take shark cartilage powder rather than capsules, you'll need to put up with a fishy odor and taste, as well as potential gastrointestinal distress including nausea, vomiting, diarrhea, and flatulence. Some patients opt to take shark cartilage enemas, but that doesn't offer much appeal either.

Safety might be an issue as well. Products made from ocean creatures, including sharks, may be contaminated with heavy metals, especially mercury. Consumers of shark cartilage may also be at risk for microbial or viral infections if the raw product is contaminated during storage and processing. Chemical contamination is also possible—chlorine is sometimes used to decrease odor and bleach the cartilage.

Given all of this information, I currently don't recommend shark cartilage even as an adjunct to conventional cancer treatment.

# Not Soy Good?

**Q:** *I hear conflicting reports about soy foods; are they healthy or harmful?*

**A:** It used to be that soy beans could do no wrong. Countless research studies have indicated that soy and soy compounds may fight cancer, protect against heart disease and osteoporosis, and offer a number of other health benefits. Now we're hearing a different story: soy may actually cause health problems. Those in the anti-soy camp claim that eating soy can cause thyroid dysfunction, mineral deficiencies, digestive disturbances, Alzheimer's disease, and even cancer. Here are the facts:

A few studies have linked soy to suppressed thyroid function; however, many experts feel that to be at risk, individuals would have to consume huge amounts of soy foods and be susceptible to hypothyroidism. If you are on thyroid medication, you do need to follow some precautions when you consume soy foods. You should always take your medication separately from any soy-based meal to avoid potential food/drug interactions. Also be aware that soybeans (and peanuts, cabbage, and some other raw plants) may act as goitrogens—compounds that interfere with the production of thyroid hormones.

Soy beans contain high levels of phytates that can bind to nutrients like calcium, iron, and zinc. Some fear that phytates may cause severe mineral deficiencies, especially in elderly populations who are at risk for malnutrition. Phytates are not unique to the soybean; they're found in the fiber-rich bran or hull of any seed, bean, nut, or other plant food. Soaking and fermenting foods can help to deactivate phytates, which is why anti-soy proponents give a thumb's up to fermented soy products like miso, natto, tamari, tempeh, and soy sauce. Before you strip your diet of all phytate-containing high fiber foods, recognize that phytates have some pretty impressive health benefits. Animal studies suggest that phytates may play a role in suppressing the growth of cancerous tumors.

According to anti-soy advocates, unfermented soy foods like soy milk, textured soy protein, and tofu contain trypsin inhibitors that prevent the breakdown of protein in the digestive tract, creating the potential for a number of digestive disturbances. These digestive enzyme "blockers" are found in all legumes, but soybeans contain the highest levels of them. Fermented foods generally have lower levels of inhibitors, but even cooked and processed soy foods like soy milk and tofu have reduced levels. While high levels of trypsin inhibitors may be harmful, low levels may have cancer-fighting properties. For individuals with digestive disturbances tied to food allergies, I suggest eating only organic soy products; genetically modified soy could contain new, unknown allergens that might trigger allergic reactions.

New research published in the *Journal of the American College of Nutrition* linked the consumption of two or more servings of tofu a week during middle age to faster brain aging, as measured by cognitive impairment and loss of brain size. Researchers for this study stressed that the connection between tofu and brain activity required further study before any implications could be drawn. Then, a study published in *Neurology* magazine noted that people in Japan, a country that consumes large amounts of tofu, had lower rates of dementia and Alzheimer's disease. Additional ongoing animal studies indicate that dietary soy protects against cognitive decline.

There is much hope in the scientific community that soy isoflavones, particularly genistein (one of the compounds found in soy), can prevent and fight cancer. A natural plant estrogen, genistein has the ability to fit into estrogen receptor sites on human cells and block the growth of hormonally induced cancers like breast, ovarian, and endometrium. Human and animal studies have shown that isoflavones can also reduce tumor size and may prevent the metastasis (spreading) of many kinds of cancer, including cancers of the prostate, lung and pancreas. However, when isoflavone consumption is high, the plant estrogen may cause a proliferation of breast cancer cells. It's too early to say for sure whether isoflavones should be used therapeutically in uterine, endometrial, ovarian, and breast cancer patients. For now, women with breast cancer (or history of a female cancer) should completely avoid dietary soy supplements and limit soy food choices to three products per week. Individuals trying to prevent cancer of any kind are encouraged to add daily servings of soy into their diet.

Nutrition experts who have reviewed the studies on the positive and adverse effects of soy feel that the benefits of soy far outweigh the risks. Until further studies help us determine appropriate levels of soy consumption, moderate intake is suggested to produce optimal health benefits. I think the easiest way to begin your "soy adventure" is to replace your regular milk with soy milk. From there, add soy nuts as a snack, try a veggie burger topped with soy cheese, and then begin cooking with tofu. You'll see lots of soy-fortified products, from pretzels to cereals; but beware—most contain very little, if any, of the active compounds.

# Sweet Poison?

**Q:** *Does sugar feed cancer?*

**A:** This is a great sound bite—sugar feeds cancer—but it's time to remove the sugar coating from this catch phrase and get to the core issue. I've talked to many people with cancer who have starved themselves while attempting to "starve" their tumors by cutting out all dietary sugars. They examine food labels and avoid breads or crackers that contain even the smallest amount of sweeteners, and they even go so far as to avoid cancer-fighting fresh fruit! It isn't easy to avoid carbohydrates, given our current food supply and lifestyle, so those individuals who succeed at following a low sugar diet have usually lost a lot of weight and are at risk for malnutrition.

I agree that high blood sugar levels are not ideal for cancer patients, or for anyone for that matter. Thankfully, our bodies produce something called insulin (or there is prescription insulin medication for people who have difficulty controlling their blood sugar) that helps to bring blood sugar levels back to normal. The more sugar you eat, the more insulin is circulated. All cells, whether they are cancerous or healthy, will accelerate their growth in response to elevated insulin levels. Furthermore, a few studies suggest that the immune system may be short circuited by a high sugar diet. Elevated blood sugar levels indirectly slow the release of growth hormones, which in turn blunt production of white blood cells. So, it does seem reasonable to assert that sugar can be detrimental for people with cancer. Ultimately, though, the goal shouldn't be to eliminate all sugars or carbohydrates, but to control blood sugar levels and hold them within a moderate range. This is the key.

You can control your blood sugar by following a few simple rules: First, to provide your body with enough energy, consume at least 50% of your daily calorie intake as carbohydrates, the majority of which should be whole grains, legumes, vegetables, and fresh fruit. These foods contain fiber, which helps to stabilize blood sugar levels and promote detoxification. Second, limit your refined sugar intake to about 5% of total calories by cutting back on the amount of obvious sweeteners in your diet, like table sugar, desserts, candies, and bakery items. Third, eat regular meals and always eat a combination of carbohydrates and protein at every meal or snack. This means including a protein source (nuts, eggs, low fat cheese, tofu, soy or whey protein powder) with fresh fruit snacks or juice on the run. Finally, read labels carefully because sweeteners tend to hide out in most processed foods. As a rule of thumb, avoid products that have sweeteners like sucrose, maltose, corn syrup, or any form of sugar listed as the first or second ingredient.

# Supplements and Surgery: A Dangerous Mix?

**Q:** *Are there any dietary supplements that I should avoid if I'm having surgery?*

**A:** As soon as you find out that you need surgery, you should have a conversation with your physician and surgeon about all the supplementary pills and powders you're taking. You may be reluctant to have this discussion, but it is in your best interest to do so. Ask specifically if there are any supplements or herbal medicines that you should avoid before or after the operation, and be sure to follow the guidelines given to you by your health care team. For more information about potential medication interactions, see www.Drugstore.com or www.Drugdigest.org. These websites feature extensive drug databases including information about drug/drug and drug/nutrient interactions.

Most doctors will tell you to stop taking your dietary supplements two to three weeks before the procedure and at least one week after surgery in order to avoid complications. Dietary supplements may cause changes in heart rate, blood pressure, or blood clotting time that could negatively impact the outcome of your surgery.

Dietary supplements that contain garlic, gingko biloba, and ginseng should be avoided at least a week before surgery. Ginseng may lower blood sugar, and all three herbs have the potential to thin the blood or interact with prescription blood thinners like Coumadin or aspirin. Vitamin E, shark cartilage, glucosamine sulfate, and fish oil may also thin the blood and increase your risk for internal bleeding.

Some supplements may interfere with, or increase, the effects of anesthesia. St. John's wort (used to treat mild depression) and valerian root (a natural sedative) should be discontinued at least two weeks before surgery. St. John's wort has been found to reduce the effects of certain drugs used before, during, and after surgery, and valerian may intensify your reaction to anesthesia.

Dietary supplements may improve your health condition, but you must do your homework before taking them. Don't try to diagnose or treat your medical condition (especially if it is a serious one) by yourself, and know the potential side effects and drug interactions of every dietary supplement you take. Remember that supplements can't replace a balanced diet, and foods rich in nutrients and protein are essential for proper wound healing and cell rebuilding after surgery.

# The New Prescription: A Tomato a Day

Q: *I've heard so much about the plant chemical lycopene. Is it really good for you and if so, what foods should I be eating to make sure I get enough in my diet?*

A: It used to be known that "an apple a day keeps the doctor away." Now, we know that tomatoes, and other lycopene-rich foods like dried apricots, guava, papaya, pink grapefruit, and watermelon may be just as beneficial when it comes to protecting our health and preventing chronic disease. Lycopene protects us because it's a powerful antioxidant that destroys free radicals that damage to cell membranes.

Some of the earliest research published on lycopene and prostate cancer came from the Harvard School of Public Health. Scientists surveyed 47,000 men regarding their eating habits over a six-year period. At the end of the study, men who consumed a diet rich in lycopene, when compared to men who consumed the lowest amount of lycopene, had a 30% lower occurrence of prostate cancer. Other studies suggest that the benefits of a "red" diet include protection against stomach and lung cancers as well.

Because the body doesn't produce lycopene, you'll need to get it through your diet. I recommend that you consume at least one serving of lycopene-rich food every day. Tomatoes and tomato products should top your list because they provide 3 to 5 mg of lycopene in just an ⅛ cup serving. An 8-ounce cup of tomato juice will provide you with 10 mg of lycopene—enough to meet the criteria for reducing your risk of prostate cancer.

While it may be tempting to consume your daily requirement of lycopene in the pill form, it is best to eat a diet containing a variety of fruits and vegetables and a combination of antioxidants—this "whole foods" approach will afford you the best protection against oxidative stress and cancer.

# Seeing Red

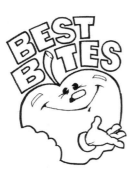

**Lycopene is fat soluble, meaning that it's best absorbed by the body if it's eaten in an oil base. Heating tomato sauce also helps the body to absorb lycopene.**

In fact, a recent study showed that lycopene is absorbed almost three times better from tomato paste than from fresh tomatoes! So, hot dishes such as chili or spaghetti sauce that include processed tomato products are among your best choices when it comes to lycopene absorption.

### Looking for lycopene?
Find it here! (per ¼ cup)

| Food Source | Lycopene, in milligrams |
| --- | --- |
| Fresh tomato | 2 mg |
| Tomato sauce | 10 mg |
| Tomato soup | 6 mg |
| Ketchup | 10 mg |
| Dried apricots | 1mg |
| Pink grapefruit | trace |
| Fresh papaya | trace |

# The Facts on Fats

Q: *I'm trying to cut back on my fat intake. Is it more important to limit satu-rated fat or partially hydrogenated fat?*

A: You'd be better off eating less of each. Just like the saturated fats found in meat, poultry, dairy, and tropical oils, hydrogenated or partially hydrogenated vegetable oils carry the same potential health risks of cancer and heart disease.

Normally, vegetable oils are good for us because they have the ability to protect our cells from toxic substances. Vegetable oils become destructive only when they are heated by high-temperature cooking methods or during the hydrogenation process. The hydrogenation process generates unnatural fats by changing the natural molecular shape of the fatty acids into abnormal "trans" shapes. There's evidence to show that trans fatty acids mutate normal cells and raise both total blood cholesterol and LDL, the "bad" cholesterol.

So why would manufacturers hydrogenate, or solidify, vegetable oils? To save time and money! Hydrogenation increases shelf life and lowers food production costs—and we end up paying the ultimate price with our health.

To cut back on trans fatty acids, be a label reader. Avoid foods that contain partially hydrogenated vegetable oils, found in rice or pasta mixes, crackers, and ready-to-eat cereals. Dairy products, processed cheeses, coffee creamers, and most margarines are chock full of trans fatty acids. If you won't give up your margarine, choose diet or whipped margarines—they contain less trans fatty acids than stick margarine. Better yet, look for Smart Balance, Spectrum, and Brummel & Brown's margarines; these spreads contain no trans fatty acids. You can also create your own healthy spread by whipping a stick of butter with a half-cup of canola or extra virgin olive oil. This "better butter," which should be stored in the refrigerator, is lower than butter in saturated fat and is relatively trans-free.

# Watch out for fractionated oils on food labels!

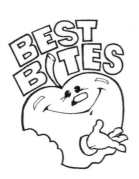

**Fractionation involves separating out the saturated fat from the oil in a particular product and then using it in place of hydrogenated fats.**

Even though fractionated oils are pretty much trans-free, they are still highly saturated, and therefore, are an unhealthy choice.

**Healthy oils that are safe to heat:**
*Canola*
*Olive*
*Grapeseed*

**Healthy oils that shouldn't be heated:**
*Flaxseed*
*Walnut*
*Hazelnut*

# Water Woes

**Q:** *Are those fancy vitamin-fortified waters I see on the supermarket shelf any good?*

**A:** It's tempting to bypass plain water for a bottle of cleverly marketed water dripping with nutrients like vitamin C and ginseng. One swig and you're on your way to better health and more energy right? Well, not exactly.

Not only do fortified bottled waters cost more than regular waters, but also, most enhanced waters contain only token amounts of nutrients. Even if your diet is unbalanced, you shouldn't look to fancy water to prevent a nutrient deficiency! If you want to supplement your diet, you should just take dietary supplements. Fortified waters containing botanicals like ginseng or echinacea also may contain less than effective amounts of these herbs to produce any health benefit—labels suggest the drink "boosts energy" or "stimulates immunity," but there is no indication as to how much of the herb has been added to the water.

If the nutrients provide few, if any, health benefits, then why are people slurping up these pricey waters? Plain and simple—they taste good! For those who are struggling to drink the suggested two to three quarts of water per day, enhanced waters seem like the perfect solution. Unfortunately, many of the waters are loaded with sugar, some contributing over 120 calories for 2½ cups of water. Other brands save on calories by sweetening the water with artificial sugars.

Because our ground water supply and streams are contaminated with pesticides, insecticides, nitrates, and other chemicals, I do believe drinking bottled water makes sense. I would choose plain bottled water, though. Filtered, chilled water does taste better than tap water and you can always add a slice of lemon or orange to enhance the flavor naturally. As bottled waters have become more popular, the Food and Drug Administration has tightened labeling regulations. Now, if the label has the word "spring" on it, then the water must come from a spring; if the water claims to be "glacial," it must come from a glacier source. Consumers should watch for misleading artwork on the labels. For example, one bottle I found was decorated with snow-capped mountains to make consumers think they're getting natural, mountain spring water, when in fact, they aren't. Finally, if you're very serious about cleaning up your water supply at home, you might want to attach a carbon filter to your kitchen faucet (remember to change often!) and eventually invest in a reverse osmosis system for your home.

# Winning at the Losing Game

**Q:** *I'm tired of diets that don't work. What are the best strategies for losing weight and keeping it off?*

**A:** Whatever your reason for losing weight—better health, more energy, or increased well being—one thing is certain: long-term weight control requires mental readiness to make dietary changes stick. Your diet plan will fail if you intend on "eating like normal" once you drop those unwanted pounds.

I believe one reason why many weight reduction diets fail is that the dieter feels a need to make too many changes all at once. I've found that most people do best if they make one dietary change at a time. Simply pick one goal—eat less sugar, drink more water, cut out all fried foods-and once you feel comfortable with those changes, introduce another dietary change and keep going until you've mastered them all! Here are some suggestions to get you started:

Change what you drink. Sugar-laden soft drinks and sports beverages should be the first to go. Replacing one 20-ounce soda with water or herbal tea can help you lose about 15 pounds of fat in a year! Try to consume at least eight, 8-ounce glasses of water throughout the day, not just in the morning or at night. This strategy will help you maintain your energy level and will promote weight loss. During the first few weeks of this weight loss plan, avoid all alcohol, which adds empty calories and relaxes your resolve to avoid mealtime splurges. Later on, establish a certain number of "no alcohol" days each week or limit alcohol to weekends and special occasions.

Eat more fruits and vegetables. There is no better way to lose weight or improve your long-term health than to eat more plants, which are naturally low in fat and calories and offer an array of health benefits. Besides containing natural chemicals that protect cells from free radical damage, fruits and vegetables contain dietary fiber. Fiber helps you feel full and stabilizes blood sugar levels—creating a slow, even energy uptake that encourages the body to use food for energy rather than storing it as body fat. Begin by eating two servings of fruit and one serving of vegetable each day. Each week, add another vegetable until you consume at least five servings of fruits and vegetables daily. Then, add a daily dose of legumes (beans, peas, or lentils) to your lunch or dinner meal.

Start eating breakfast. If you eat something every morning, you can help stave off hunger pangs that lead to overeating later on in the day. This is particularly true if you eat a protein-based breakfast, which helps to keep your blood sugar levels in check. Try these quick a.m. energizers: add nuts to a cup of yogurt, eat a hard boiled egg with toast, or drink a soy and fruit smoothie on your way out the door in the morning.

Eat the right kind of fats. Use extra virgin olive or canola oil most often. Try to eat fish at least once a week and start sprinkling ground flax seed on top of oatmeal or salad greens. Researchers have shown that coldwater fish (salmon, tuna, mackerel, and others) contain health-promoting omega-3 fatty acids that promote weight loss by regulating insulin metabolism. Work toward reducing the amount of partially hydrogenated, or hydrogenated oils (found in almost every convenience food item) you consume by cooking from scratch more often.

Eat better, fast. Steer clear of hamburgers, deep fried fish, or breaded chicken sandwiches served at local fast food joints. Instead, choose a broiled chicken sandwich (minus the mayo) or a BK Veggie Burger, which offers on-the-run diners a tasty, grain- and vegetable-filled alternative to beef. Don't be tempted to top it with cheese, unless you want an extra 9 grams of fat. Chinese take-out can also be a dieter's downfall. Did you know that a typical order of Kung Pao chicken contains as much fat as four Quarter Pounders? You can cut the fat off many Asian entrées by keeping to the 1:1 rule: one cup entree to one cup rice. And finally, the best rule to follow when dining out at fast food restaurants: Never, ever say "supersize!"

Plan for a food vacation day. Every once in a while, you know you're going to go "off" your regular, healthy meal plan, so don't beat yourself up about it. What you do most often will impact your long-term health. Commit to five days of healthful eating, and then allow yourself a favorite indulgence once a week. This will help you from feeling deprived. After your off day, balance out the excessive calorie and fat intake by going vegetarian for the day—replace all meats, eggs, dairy foods, and butter with platefuls of fruits, vegetables, whole grains, beans, and nuts.

Shape your body. The latest scientific findings suggest that for permanent weight loss, aerobic exercises should be complemented with resistance training. Lifting weights burns fat and can increase muscle mass, making it progressively easier every week for the body to burn more calories. Begin by lifting soup cans or invest in handheld dumb bells—and if you can, start your mornings with ten minutes of resistance exercises. A number of studies show that exercising early in the morning helps you burn calories all day long. Eventually, move into a three- or four-day routine of low intensity, aerobic exercise combined with a fifteen-minute muscle building weight lifting session. Please remember, it's important to get clearance from your medical doctor before you begin an exercise program.

# Try, and succeed!

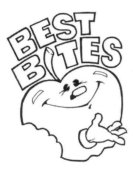

**Scientists know that dropping extra weight reduces risk of disease and death. But now we have evidence that just attempting to lose weight might lower your mortality rate!**

The United States Centers for Disease Control and Prevention reported that individuals who were overweight and tried to lose weight but failed, still reduced their risk of early death! Researchers suggest that perhaps any attempt to lose weight might tie into other behaviors that can lower mortality.

*This news gives new meaning to the saying "Think thin"!*

**How to trim 100 calories:**
- Split a bag of small fries with a friend
- Eat two servings of nonfat dairy foods in place of regular dairy foods
- Use one teaspoon mustard in place of one tablespoon regular mayonnaise
- Don't add cream to your morning coffee and take a 15-minute walk

# Index

cocoa 26–27
coffee 6, 16, 38–39, 72, 114
colon therapy 21, 40
coral calcium 32–33
coumadin 30, 36, 37, 103
cyanotoxins 67

### • D •

DDT 53
deep vein thrombosis 36
deodorized garlic supplements 59
dessicated liver 73
detoxification 17, 19, 20, 24, 39–40, 62,
    66, 75, 81, 91, 102
diabetes 17, 23, 32, 38, 73, 81
dietary optimists 21
dietary supplements
    before surgery 103–104
    calcium 15, 16, 32
    CoQ10  19
    deodorized garlic 59
    during cancer treatment 19–20
    folic acid 9
    garlic 58–59
    green foods 37, 57
    iron 73, 90
    N-acetyl cysteine 19
    risks of 31, 44
    vitamin E 20, 62, 73, 103
    whole foods 57
digestive enzymes 3, 4, 9, 28, 29, 40, 41,
    99
drug/nutrient interactions 31, 103

### • E •

energy bars 43–44
    recommended brands 44
erucic acid 21–22
Essiac tea 47–48

### • F •

fasting 39, 75
fat substitutes 49–50
fats
    essential 45–46, 50–51
    monounsaturated 22, 170
    omega-3 12, 13, 18, 30, 45, 46, 51,
        54, 55, 60, 70
    polyunsaturated 70
    saturated 13, 18, 87, 107–108
fiber
    food sources of  9, 10, 11–12, 17,
        40, 63, 98, 102, 112
    lignans 51, 62
    NCI recommendations for 17
fish 3, 5, 14, 18, 45, 53–54, 55, 70, 112
fish oil 37, 46, 55, 103
flavonoids 70
flax 6, 14, 18, 73, 108, 112
Flor-essence 48
folic acid 9, 21
food allergy 3, 99
food combining diet 28–29
food intolerances (see also food sensitivi-
    ties) 3, 4, 42
free range 83

### • G •

garlic 58–59
genetically modified foods 22, 60–61
genistein 199, 99
glucosamine sulfate 103
glycemic index 23
goitrogens 98
green foods supplements 37, 57
grilled meats 68–69

### • H •

hardening of the arteries 38, 40, 65, 66
healthy diet on a budget 34–35
heart disease 9, 12, 13, 17, 18, 26, 32,
    54, 60, 73, 81, 94, 98, 107

## • P •

PCB 53, 55
pesticides 53, 60, 74, 83–84, 110
pH 1–2
phytates 15, 98, 99
phytochemicals 17
phytoestrogens 61
plasticizers 85–86
plastics 85
PMS 45
polycyclic aromatic hydrocarbons 68
polyphenols 64, 65, 94
prebiotic 88
probiotics 42, 59, 87–88
produce 56–57
produce washes 84

## • R •

radiation 3, 19, 48, 54, 67, 75, 92
rapeseed (see canola) 21, 22, 60
raw foods diet 91–92
reishi mushroom 81–82
reverse osmosis 110

## • S •

saponins 66
sarcoidosis 16
saturated fat 13, 18, 87, 107–108
shark cartilage 31, 96–97
shiitake mushroom 70, 81–82
soy 9, 19, 24, 35, 43, 60, 61, 77, 89,
  98–100
sprouts 35, 66, 93
Stevia 8, 27
sugar
  alternatives 7, 8
  and cancer 101–102
  curbing intake 23–25
  health complications from 23
surgery, supplements to stop before
  103–104

## • T •

tea
  black 65
  green 26, 33, 36, 64–65, 70
  herbal 65, 111
  Essiac 57–48
tofu 77, 89, 99, 100, 102
tomato 105–106
trans fatty acids 13, 18, 23, 107–108
triglycerides 45
trypsin inhibitors 99

## • V •

vitamin C – food sources 72
vitamins
  B6  9, 19
  B12  9, 73, 90
  C  15, 72, 73, 81
  D  16
  E  20, 62, 73, 103
  folic acid 9
  K  36–37
  multivitamin 78–79

## • W •

water
  bottled 109–110
  vitamin fortified 109
weight gain 5, 7, 23
weight loss 24, 29, 70, 111–113
whey protein 6, 75, 102
whole grains 62–63

## • Y •

yogurt 42, 59, 87–88
  frozen 87

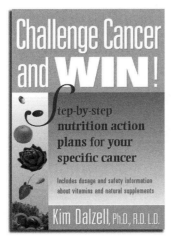